# Introduction to Horse Nutrition

# Dedication

This book is dedicated to my ever supportive husband and family, and to my mum Ricky – a true inspiration to all who knew her, but particularly to me.

# Introduction to Horse Nutrition

Zoe Davies MSc RNutr

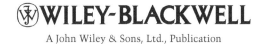

A John Wiley & Sons, Ltd., Publication

This edition first published 2009
© 2009 by Zoe Davies

Blackwell Publishing was acquired by John Wiley & Sons in February 2007.
Blackwell's publishing programme has been merged with Wiley's global Scientific,
Technical, and Medical business to form Wiley-Blackwell.

*Registered office*
John Wiley & Sons Ltd, The Atrium, Southern Gate, Chichester, West Sussex,
PO19 8SQ, United Kingdom

*Editorial offices*
9600 Garsington Road, Oxford, OX4 2DQ, United Kingdom
2121 State Avenue, Ames, Iowa 50014-8300, USA

For details of our global editorial offices, for customer services and for information
about how to apply for permission to reuse the copyright material in this book please
see our website at www.wiley.com/wiley-blackwell.

*Library of Congress Cataloging-in-Publication Data*

Davies, Zoe.
   Introduction to horse nutrition / Zoe Davies.
       p.   ;   cm.
   Includes bibliographical references and index.
   ISBN 978-1-4051-6998-1 (pbk. : alk. paper)   1. Horses–Nutrition–
Requirements.   2. Horses–Feeding and feeds.   I. Title.
   [DNLM:   1. Animal Nutritional Physiological Phenomena.   2. Horses.   3. Animal
Feed.   4. Animal Husbandry–methods.   5. Diet–veterinary.   SF 285.5 D257i 2009]
   SF285.5.D38 2009
   636.1'0852–dc22

                                                                    2009005457

A catalogue record for this book is available from the British Library.

Set in 10/13pt Palatino by SNP Best-set Typesetter Ltd., Hong Kong

1   2009

# Contents

# A Reader's Perspective

*Introduction to Horse Nutrition* provides practical information on horse diet and nutrition, and the effect it has on health and performance. The importance of nutrition cannot be underestimated as horses are entirely dependent upon the trainer or owner's feeding management and choices. Poor nutrition is common and while deficiencies may initially result in minor ailments they can ultimately become factors in the development of cancer and other degenerative diseases. Inadequate nutrition and unnatural diets also have an adverse affect on horse behaviour and their ability to cope with stress. Furthermore, horses are all individuals and their nutritional requirements are subject to genetic make-up, age, gender, diets present and past, environment and other factors. Demand for reliable and instructive information regarding horse nutrition has never been greater and Zoe provides this with great success in this highly relevant book

We have been breeding and racing horses for many years at Boxhedge Hall Stud. Zoe has undertaken the nutritional management for the past twenty years, and doubtless her skill and knowledge have contributed to our many successes at Group level, including Tomba winning the Prix de la Foret and the Cork and Orrery Stakes; Holding Court, winner of the Prix du Jockey Club; Consular, winner of the Old Newton Cup; Ordnance Row, winner of the Sovereign Stakes and Delegator, winner of the Craven Stakes and runner up of the 2009 Two Thousand Guineas, to name but a few.

This is a small team operation and so attention to detail is vital. Zoe has helped the team to efficiently manage diet and nutrition for all the horses, resulting in optimal strength and performance over their racing and breeding careers. Zoe ensures that Boxhedge Stud remains at the forefront of current equine nutritional practice.

As well as having over 25 years of experience in the field, Zoe is registered with the Nutrition Society of Great Britain, an honour only granted to those with a substantial level of experience and expertise. Zoe is highly qualified, both technically and practically to write this important book and, in my opinion, it should be read by *everyone* who feeds horses.

**Poilin Good – Owner/Breeder – Boxhedge Hall Stud**

# Introduction

*… A horse is a thing of such beauty …*
*None will tire of looking at him*
*As long as he displays himself in his splendour*
**Xenophon 400** BC

The subject of horse nutrition is often misunderstood. There are numerous old wives' tales and mystical concoctions and formulas to be found in feed rooms around the world some of which are quite detrimental to horses' health. This often quite technical subject justifiably confuses many students and horse owners. Nutrition has long been recognised as a vital and integral part of horse care and is known to be important for horse health, reproduction, performance and general well being. This book, although it is aimed at all students of horse management, is equally important for horse owners or those wishing to learn more about equine nutrition. Malnutrition of horses is unfortunately widespread, mostly due to misinformation and confusion. The vast array of commercial products available for feeding to horses does not help this situation, and overfeeding and over-supplementation with resulting health and performance problems are becoming more common. Nutrition is the fuel that keeps the equine machine running efficiently. Horses are healthier, happier and more likely to perform at their best when given the correct balance of nutrients to do so. There are many horses and ponies that could have significantly improved health and athletic and breeding performance if fed properly, according to their physiological and psychological needs.

The aim of this book is to *introduce* the subject of horse nutrition to all students and horse owners at a level that is easy to understand. The first part of the book covers the often complex subject of biological molecules and the basic chemistry of nutrition for students.

In 2007 the 6th edition of the NRC *Nutrient Requirements of Horses* was published after a long wait. This provides the latest data for nutrient requirements and is often referred to throughout the text.

# The Horse as a Herbivore

Food is the material ingested by horses; it is then broken down into its constituent parts during the process of digestion before being absorbed into the body for use. Essential nutrients are the chemical substances in food, which cannot be made in sufficient amounts by the horse itself. These substances are required for life and growth and work.

Various foods contain different nutrients that are used within the horse's body in different ways. The growth of a foal into an adult horse requires important building blocks provided by many different nutrients, as does the production of milk by a lactating mare. For muscles to work and move the horse forward (or sideways or backward!), they must be supplied with energy giving nutrients. The horse needs nutrients to move, work, reproduce, breathe and lactate.

Horses, like all living organisms, need to take in substances in order to make new cells and tissues, repair old ones or release energy. This is known as nutrition or feeding.

The nutrients in the natural diet of the horse are supplied mostly by herbage such as grass. Grass is a green plant and all green plants are able to take in simple substances such as water, carbon dioxide and nitrogen (in the form of nitrate or ammonia) and inorganic minerals and build them into more complex organic substances such as carbohydrates and proteins.

Green plants are able to harness the energy from the sun combining it with other chemical elements to provide complex organic substances. These organic substances made by plants provide nutrients for animals grazing upon them (Figure 1.1). Plants make carbohydrates from carbon dioxide and water using energy from sunlight. This process is called *photosynthesis* and takes place in the leaves of all green plants. Plant leaves could therefore be considered as carbohydrate factories.

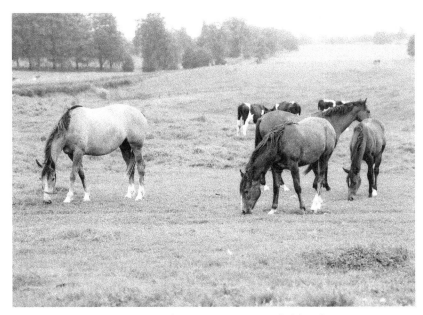

**Figure 1.1**   Horses grazing, taking in nutrients provided by plants.

The balanced chemical equation for photosynthesis is:

$$6CO_2 + \underset{\text{chlorophyll (green plants)}}{\overset{\text{sunlight}}{6H_2O}} \rightarrow C_6H_{12}O_6 + 6O_2$$

The carbohydrates produced by photosynthesis are either used straight away or converted into substances that provide structural support to the plant cells. Any remaining are stored as complex carbohydrates. Most of the carbohydrates though are made into supporting tissues to maintain the structural cell walls. The cell walls are made up of a fibre matrix of cellulose with hemicellulose and lignin (see Chapter 3). Plants are therefore able to feed themselves, a process known as *autotrophic* nutrition.

Horses similar to all other animals have a limited ability to make their own carbohydrates although they can make lactose and glycogen. In their simplest form, carbohydrates such as glucose are soluble so they can be transported around the horse's body to the tissues where they are needed. Here, they are oxidised back to carbon dioxide and water by the process of respiration, which releases the energy for cellular processes.

Horses must feed or take in the organic substances described above that are originally manufactured by green plants. This is known as *heterotrophic* nutrition. Horses are herbivores and so eat green plants, mostly grass with a large proportion of leaf.

## DIET

Everything horses eat and drink daily is known as the *diet*. A diet that contains all the nutrients in the correct proportions is known as a *balanced diet*. A *ration* is the food allowance for one day supplied to the horse; it may have been previously evaluated by the horse owner. A *feedstuff* is any material used as food.

Complex molecules such as carbohydrates, fats and proteins are required to provide energy and other materials for growth, repair, movement and general life functions of the horse. These are known as macronutrients. Other nutrients such as vitamins and minerals are required in much smaller amounts and these are called micronutrients.

Horses need the following essential nutrients in the diet:

- Carbohydrates
- Fats (lipids)
- Proteins (amino acids)
- Vitamins
- Minerals (inorganic elements)
- Water (not actually classified as a nutrient).

Malnutrition results from an unbalanced diet where some nutrients are deficient or completely lacking. In addition, over-supply of some nutrients such as carbohydrates may result in ill health or chronic problems such as insulin resistance and laminitis.

Individual horses have different nutrient needs depending upon age, height, workload, stage of life, and breed and external factors such as temperature.

## EVOLUTION

The horse evolved to roam grasslands foraging on fibrous grasses, weeds and occasional browsing of small bushes. Extensive fossil records have revealed the evolutionary pathway of *Equus*. This was not a straight evolutionary line, but a sort of tree shaped evolution with many dead ends resulting in the loss of that particular ancestor of the modern horse (see Figure 1.2).

Horses can be traced back to the Eocene period 50–60 million years ago, to a small fox like animal known as *Hyracotherium* (also referred to as dawn horse or Eohippus) (Figure 1.3). This small animal weighed around 5 kilograms (12 pounds). In the Miocene period, approximately

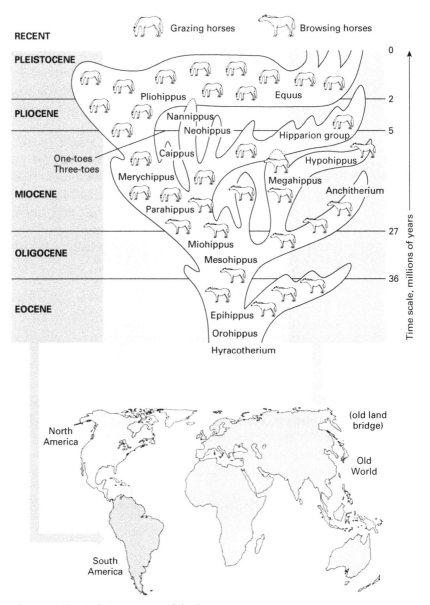

**Figure 1.2** Evolutionary tree of the horse.

27 million years ago, many of the horse's ancestors moved away from the tropical swampy forests they inhabited on to the plains in order to survive, although some remained behind to carry on living in the forests. This was due to changes in the global climate producing drier grasslands and plains. Changes in the genetic makeup over a long

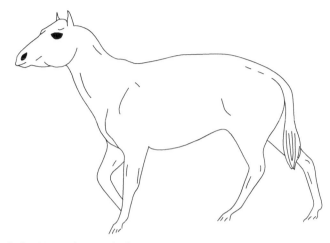

**Figure 1.3**  Hyracotherium (Eohippus, Dawn Horse).

period of time helped these ancestors to adapt to their new grazing diets. Grass plant cells contain cellulose within the cell walls, a complex carbohydrate which is basically indigestible to all mammals including horses unless they develop some way of breaking down the cellulose to unlock the nutrients contained within.

Grass also contains silica, which is an extremely hard substance and so grazing horses would need to evolve teeth capable of withstanding the grinding of herbage containing silica and also the frequent presence of soil particles attached to the grass. This was a 'gritty' diet! The head became bigger in order to house the longer grinding teeth. The jaw increased in depth to house more powerful muscles for 'grinding'. To this end, the jaws became sideways moving to more efficiently break down and tear the fibrous food. Teeth also became coated with cement and became higher crowned or *hypsodont*. Eventually these teeth undertook continuous growth or *hypselodont*. The neck became longer to allow the animal to reach down and graze. The limbs also became longer allowing them to run faster away from predators.

The digestive system also evolved in several ways to adapt to the diet. In order to break down cellulose many herbivores have adopted a symbiotic arrangement with millions of microbes in their guts which are able to produce an enzyme, namely cellulase, which breaks down cellulose contained in plant cell walls. The horse in turn provides a safe environment in which the microbes can live in a specialised digestive area. Most herbivores therefore evolved large fermentation areas within the gut in which the millions of bacteria live and ferment the ingested plant material anaerobically (i.e. in the absence of oxygen).

The ruminant stomach developed into a large multi-compartmented section of the digestive tract known as the fore stomachs. Perhaps the most well known of these is the rumen, but the reticulum, omasum and abomasum also support fermentation. The fore stomachs are situated between the oesophagus and the small intestine. Horses, however (and rabbits, tapirs and rhinoceroses), have developed an exceptionally large fermentation area (caecum) within the large intestine or hindgut, following the simple stomach and small intestine (see Figure 1.4). Ruminants are consequently known as foregut cranial fermentors, or pregastric digesters or fermentors and horses as hindgut caudal fermentors, or postgastric fermentors.

The basic breakdown of cellulose in the rumen and caecum is essentially the same, however the position of the fermentation area relative to the small intestine has implications for the amount of nutrients absorbed. The small intestine is the only part of the digestive tract that allows simple carbohydrates and amino acids, the products of breakdown by digestive enzymes secreted by the horse, to be absorbed. For horses, sugars and dietary starch are broken down by enzymes within the small intestine and absorbed. Ruminants, however, ferment sugars and starch within the fore stomachs.

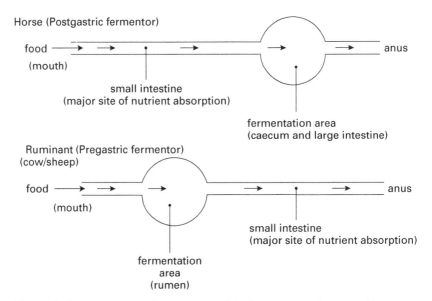

**Figure 1.4** Comparison of the position of the foregut in ruminants and horses.

Dead and dying bacteria from the rumen are passed into the true stomach and small intestine of the ruminant where they are further digested and component nutrients are utilised by the ruminant (Figure 1.5). Thus ruminants are able to use microbial protein whereas microbial protein produced in the hindgut of the horse is largely wasted. Therefore the ruminant is more efficient at digesting forage than the horse. A comparison of nutrition in ruminants and horses is shown in Table 1.1.

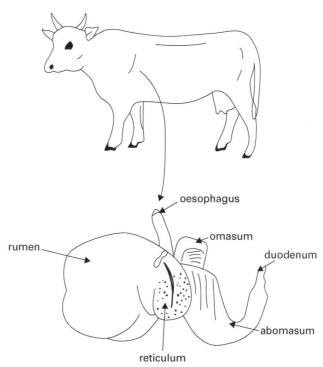

**Figure 1.5**   The forestomachs of the ruminant.

**Table 1.1**   Comparison of equine and ruminant nutrition.

| Digestive function | Horses | Ruminants |
|---|---|---|
| Remove energy from plant cellulose through fermentation | √ | √ |
| Use dietary sugars directly | √ | X |
| Break down microbial material for further nutrients in small intestine | X | √ |

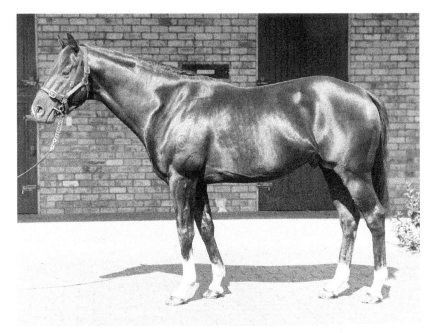

**Figure 1.6**  A horse in excellent condition. (Courtesy Jo Prestwich)

The caecum and colon must retain digesta (food swallowed for digestion) for a long time to give the microbial population time to break down the fibre.

Essentially the physiology of the digestive tract of the modern day horse is exactly the same as that of its ancestors, which developed the ability to ferment complex carbohydrates from herbage via a hindgut fermentation chamber.

The practice of feeding horses and the nutrients required are at all times based upon this principle in order to maintain the health of both the digestive tract and the horse itself. Horses receiving optimal nutrition visibly appear in excellent condition (Figure 1.6).

**Summary points**

- Essential nutrients are the chemical substances in food that cannot be made in sufficient amounts by the horse itself.
- Green plants are able to harness the energy from the sun combining it with other chemical elements to provide complex organic substances.
- Everything horses eat and drink daily is known as the *diet*.
- A diet that contains all the nutrients in the correct proportions is known as a *balanced diet*.
- Macronutrients are complex molecules such as carbohydrates, fats and proteins that are required to provide energy and other materials for growth, repair, movement and general life functions of the horse.
- Micronutrients are required in much smaller amounts, for example vitamins and minerals.
- The horse's digestive system evolved to adapt to the forage diet. In order to break down cellulose, many herbivores have adopted a symbiotic arrangement with millions of bacteria in their guts.
- Essentially the physiology of the digestive tract of the modern day horse is exactly the same as that of its ancestors which developed the ability to ferment complex carbohydrates from herbage via a hindgut fermentation chamber.

# Structure and Function of the Equine Digestive System

Horses are herbivores consuming huge quantities of roughage containing a high proportion of cellulose (found in plant cell walls) while grazing. Horses although technically grazers will also browse hedges and small trees if available. Horses are classed as simple stomached or monogastric, similar to pigs and humans. Horses cannot produce the enzyme cellulase, which is required to break down cellulose. Instead, horses have developed a huge store of microbes or microorganisms in the hindgut (large intestine and caecum) that produce cellulase and are therefore able to break down cellulose to energy producing substances known as volatile fatty acids. These microorganisms use some of the substances produced such as proteins for their own growth thereby helping the colonies to survive in the hindgut environment. Some of the products of bacterial fermentation are then absorbed by the caecum. Following breakdown of the food and removal of the nutrients from the gut, the remainder is excreted as waste.

Parts of the horse's digestive system are sacculated which is thought to reduce the flow of food through it. The digestive system is the collective name used to describe the alimentary canal and accessory organs associated with it such as the pancreas. The alimentary canal begins at the mouth, passes through the thorax, abdomen and pelvis and ends at the anus. The alimentary canal is the long tube through which food passes. It can take as long as 72 hours for fibrous food to pass through the horse's digestive system.

The digestive system of the horse is unique and can be split into two parts:

- Foregut – stomach and small intestine (duodenum, jejunum, ileum)
- Hindgut – caecum, large colon, small colon and rectum.

The horse's digestive tract is shown in Figure 2.1.

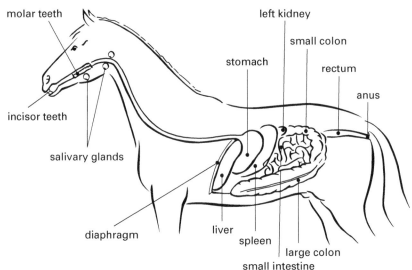

**Figure 2.1**   Foregut and hindgut of the horse.

## Foregut

The foregut is very similar to that of humans and pigs. The hindgut is similar to the rumen of a cow or a sheep, i.e. it is where the vast majority of fermentation takes place.

The foregut consists of the mouth, pharynx, oesophagus, stomach and small intestine. The hindgut consists of the caecum, large colon, small colon, rectum and anus. The horse's digestive tract is approximately 30 m (100 ft) long and in order to fit into the abdominal space it is long and looped and loosely held in place by sheets of connective tissue known as the mesentery. The digestive tract as seen from below is shown in Figure 2.2.

## Teeth

Equine teeth differ from human ones in that they grow continually throughout the life of the horse (Figure 2.3). This is due to the constant grinding action that wears down the molars.

The horse has two sets of teeth during its lifetime:

- Temporary – whiter
- Permanent – more yellow.

There are no temporary molars, as the jaw of the young horse does not have enough space. From the age of 2.5 years the milk teeth are

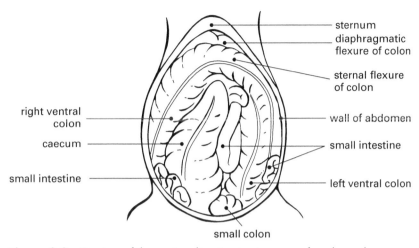

**Figure 2.2**  Structure of the equine digestive tract, as seen from beneath.

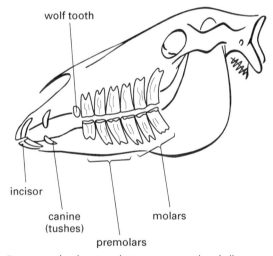

**Figure 2.3**  Equine teeth, showing their position in the skull.

gradually replaced and most horses have a full set of permanent teeth by five years of age and these last the lifetime of the horse.

The adult horse has three types of teeth:

- Incisors – biting teeth
- Molars – grinding teeth
- Canines – tushes.

In horses only a small part of the crown is visible above the gum line but the tooth grows continuously upwards to compensate for the grinding action and therefore erosion of teeth while chewing.

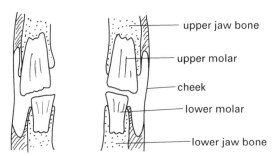

**Figure 2.4**   The upper jaw is slightly wider than the lower jaw.

Each tooth contains three layers:

• Dentine – calcium-containing substance in the centre of the tooth
• Enamel – porcelain which is a very hard substance that covers the crown
• Cement – covers the crown to provide further strength.

The grinding action of teeth is vital to break down the fibrous food. To this end the upper jaw is slightly wider than the lower jaw creating a shearing action when chewing (Figure 2.4). This can create sharp edges over time, which must be filed to prevent the mouth becoming sore from the sharp teeth, which can stop horses eating. Horses with poor teeth may be quidding, i.e. dropping half chewed food out of the mouth when eating. The teeth of older horses can become loose and weak and this can result in reduced food intake. The care of old horses' teeth is vital and if they are no longer able to chew long fibre efficiently, feed should be soaked with short, soft chaffs to provide a mash.

## Mouth

Horses have strong sensitive and mobile lips (*labia oris*) enabling them to sort through food and graze close to the ground (Figure 2.5). The incisors break off the food and the lips pass this on to the tongue. The horse's tongue is important for the movement of food within the mouth. Water and milk are drawn into the mouth by suction caused by a negative pressure in the mouth, created largely by the action of the tongue.

From here material is ground down by the molars through a series of chewing movements (side to side and up and down). The action of chewing is also known as mastication. Horses chew many more times when eating forage compared to concentrate feed. While chewing,

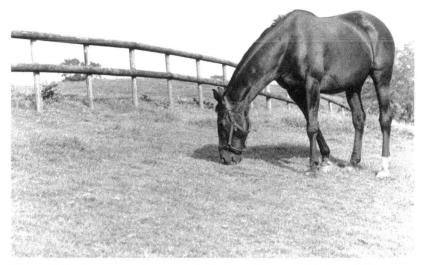

**Figure 2.5**  Horses crop the grass with incisors. (Courtesy of Jo Prestwich)

saliva is produced and this acts as a lubricant before swallowing. The mixture of food and saliva that is swallowed is then known as chyme. The act of swallowing is known as deglutition. Saliva is produced by three sets of salivary glands situated on the sides of the face. Horses have three pairs of salivary glands (Figure 2.6):

- Parotid (largest salivary gland found near the poll)
- Submaxillary (found in the jaw)
- Sublingual (found under the tongue).

The parotid glands are roughly 20 cm long and 2 cm wide with an average weight of about 200 g. The submaxillary and sublingual glands are much smaller. The ducts from each gland empty into the cavity of the mouth where saliva is secreted. The presence of food in the mouth and chewing stimulate saliva production in horses; it is not produced in anticipation of food as in some animals, such as dogs. Saliva in horses has no digestive activity as it does not contain salivary amylase which begins digestion of starch, however it does contain bicarbonate to help neutralise the acid in the horse's stomach. The buffering capacity of equine saliva is thought to be much less than that in ruminants. Dry food results in the secretion of more watery saliva. High fibre diets

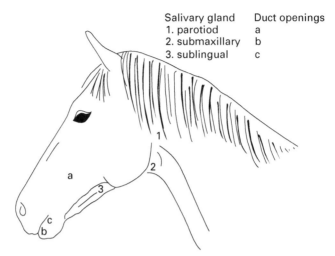

Salivary gland    Duct openings
1. parotiod          a
2. submaxillary   b
3. sublingual      c

**Figure 2.6**  Horses have three pairs of salivary glands.

yield more saliva as more chewing occurs resulting in more bicarbonate for buffering of stomach acid and it is thought that a 500 kg horse on a forage only diet may secrete up to 25 litres per day.

As food is eaten, it is ground down by chewing and mixed with saliva before forming a bolus at the back of the mouth, which is then swallowed.

The action of swallowing occurs when the highly muscular tongue pushes the bolus of food to the back of the mouth, towards the pharynx. The food passes into the pharynx and down the oesophagus. The pharynx is a muscular funnel roughly 15 cm long, which belongs to both the digestive and respiratory passages. Food is quickly swallowed so that it will not enter the nasal passages or larynx, which is protected by the epiglottis as food passes through. The epiglottis, a small flap of cartilage that forms part of the larynx, moves upwards and forwards to cover the trachea (windpipe) preventing food entering the airways.

## Oesophagus

This is a muscular tube about 1.2 to 1.5 m long extending down the left side of the neck leading from the pharynx to the stomach; it is the first main organ of digestion. Solid food moves down the oesophagus by waves of muscular contractions known as peristalsis whereas liquids are thought to be squirted down. Muscle fibres in the oesophagus contract and relax in turn creating a wave of movement pushing the food known as the bolus down the oesophagus. This movement is one way only, i.e. downwards towards the stomach. The lining of the oesophagus secretes mucus to aid passage to the stomach. Occasionally food becomes lodged or stuck in the oesophagus and this is known as choke (see Chapter 12).

## Stomach

The stomach is a 'U' shaped elastic organ, which is relatively small compared with the overall size of the horse and has a capacity of 10–13 litres and is about the size of a rugby ball; the rumen of the cow may hold ten times as much. Food enters the stomach from the oesophagus through a valve known as the cardiac sphincter. The purpose of this valve is to stop the stomach contents moving back into the oesophagus and therefore horses are unable to vomit or belch. Pressure can build up within the stomach to such an extent that the stomach may rupture. Food leaves the stomach through another valve known as the pyloric sphincter and enters the duodenum, the first part of the small intestine. Owing to the shape of the stomach, the entrance and exit are quite close to one another and this also allows water to pass over food in the main part of the stomach because of its U shape.

The wall of the stomach consists of muscular layers with an inner mucous membrane. The horse's stomach is unique in that it has two distinct regions with quite different characteristics. The upper one third of the stomach is termed the *saccus caecus* and is the squamous or non-glandular stomach, anatomically similar to the oesophagus. The inner surface of the mucosa is made up of layers of flat cells known as squamous cells, which line the area of the *saccus caecus* and are susceptible to damage by stomach acid because of the lack of mucus as there are no mucus producing cells in this region. The bottom two thirds of the stomach is termed the glandular or non-squamous stomach and this lines the fundic and pyloric regions of the stomach. This area is composed of a number of cell types that are responsible for the initial digestion of food and this includes mucus, hydrochloric acid and pepsinogen – the precursor of pepsin. The pH of this area of the stomach is very low due to the production of acid. The 'junction' between the two distinct areas is known as the *margo plicatus* (Figure 2.7)

Functions of the stomach include:

- Begins protein digestion through the action of enzymes
- Mixes food with gastric juices
- Lubricates food by secreting mucus
- Kills bacteria by secreting hydrochloric acid.

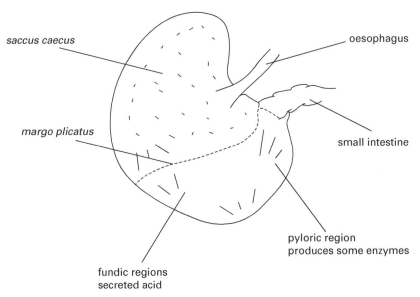

saccus caecus

oesophagus

margo plicatus

small intestine

pyloric region
produces some enzymes

fundic regions
secreted acid

**Figure 2.7** Structure of the equine stomach.

The horse has evolved as a trickle feeder eating small amounts often, the stomach is only a temporary holding vessel in horses. Food begins to break down in the stomach due to enzymic activity and some microbial digestion of soluble carbohydrates also takes place in the less acidic regions. However, there is only a small amount of fibre digestion in the stomach as fermentation produces gas, which would cause pain, as horses do not belch. Microbes may be found in all areas of the stomach, but the majority seem to be found in the *saccus caecus*. Further microbial populations are found in the fundic region and these may produce VFAs (volatile fatty acids) and lactic acid.

As the food distends the stomach, the hormone gastrin is produced which stimulates production of gastric juice by the fundic glands. Some 10–30 l of gastric juice is secreted daily by the stomach and this contains:

- Hydrochloric acid – produced by parietal cells, it neutralises bacteria and activates pepsin
- Pepsinogen (pepsin precursor) – an enzyme that acts on protein to produce peptones to begin digestion
- Gastric lipase – present in very small amounts, it helps to reduce fats to fatty acids and glycerol, minimal action
- Rennin (foals only) curdles milk.

Gastric juice is produced continuously in horses although the rate of secretion varies. Digesta or chyme (food once in the digestive system) is kept within the stomach for a relatively short time usually around 20 minutes or so before passing into the small intestine. This suits the horse's natural trickle feeding pattern of little and often.

## Small intestine

The length of the small intestine in the horse is relatively short at approximately 21–25 m with a capacity of 55–70 l depending upon the size of the horse. The small intestine of the cow is much longer at around 40 m. The small intestine runs from the stomach to the caecum and is split into three parts:

* Duodenum (approximately 1 m)
* Jejunum (approximately 20 m)
* Ileum (approximately 1.5 m).

The pancreatic and bile ducts enter the duodenum roughly 15 cm from the stomach. There are three types of glands in the small intestine namely:

* Crypts of Lieberkuhn – intestinal glands
* Bruner's glands – duodenal glands
* Peyer's patches.

The pH of digesta entering the small intestine from the acidic stomach is quite low at 2.5–3.5. Bile and the secretion of bicarbonate from Bruner's glands in the duodenum then raise the pH by buffering the acid to pH7–7.5 which creates a more beneficial environment for the function of digestive enzymes and the absorption of nutrients across the intestinal wall.

The inner wall of the small intestine is covered with tiny finger-like projections (0.5–1 mm in length) known as villi. Thess increase the surface area for improved absorption and contain a network of blood capillaries and lymph vessels. At the base of the villi lie the Crypts of Lieberkuhn, which secrete mucus and some enzymes to cover the surface of the intestine. Digestive enzymes are also secreted by the pancreas.

The main function of the small intestine is to complete digestion of simple carbohydrates (sugar and starch), lipids (fats and oils), amino acids, vitamins and minerals. The end products are then absorbed via the villi into blood capillaries. Most absorption takes place in the jejunum. Digestion and absorption take place in the small intestine as peristaltic movements mix the food with intestinal and pancreatic juices and bile. Recent research has shown the presence of some microbes that break down cellulose within the duodenum although there are fewer than in the stomach. Starch digestion is a three-step process, which begins with the action of the enzyme pancreatic amylase, however horses are not well adapted to digest large amounts of dietary starch. The amount of α-amylase is variable and much lower than in animals with simple stomachs such as pigs and humans. Cereal starch should therefore be processed by cooking, micronising, steaming, and so on to help increase starch digestibility and only small amounts should be given in each feed. Horses are able to digest sugars very well.

Glucose is absorbed by both facilitative and passive transport:

- Facilitative transport – carrier proteins transport nutrients into cells of the intestinal wall down a concentration gradient, i.e. from an area of high concentration to low concentration
- Passive transport – nutrients simply diffuse across the intestinal wall down a concentration gradient from an area of high concentration to low concentration.

Nutrients may also be absorbed by active transport, a more complicated process whereby the nutrient is carried across the intestinal barrier attached to a complex protein and either a hydrogen or sodium ion.

Some nutrients are absorbed by a process called pinocytosis where intestinal cells actually surround nutrients and 'pinch' them into the intestinal cell. This is common in foals.

Table 2.1 Shows the enzymic processes that occur in the foregut.

Fat soluble vitamins A, D, E and K are absorbed with fats via active transport and passive diffusion. Mineral absorption also occurs including calcium, phosphorus, potassium, chloride, zinc and copper.

Bile is secreted by the liver and is a product of the breakdown of red blood cells. It is greenish yellow in colour and contains salts, bile pigments (bilirubin and biliverdin), acids and water. Bile not only helps to neutralise the acid from the stomach but also emulsifies fats turning them into smaller droplets for action by enzymes. Unlike humans, the horse does not have a gall bladder in which to store bile, instead bile trickles continuously into the duodenum from the liver via the bile duct. This is because horses are not 'meal' eaters; their digestive systems have evolved to eat little and often, and mostly highly fibrous material.

The rate of passage of food through the small intestine is relatively fast and food will reach the caecum in just over one hour. Non-fibrous

**Table 2.1**  Enzymic processes in the foregut.

| Origin | Enzyme | Substrate | End product of digestion |
|---|---|---|---|
| **Stomach** | | | |
| Body chief cells | Pepsin | Proteins | Proteoses, peptones |
| Fundic neck chief cells | Gastric lipase | Fats | Fatty acids, glycerol |
| **Pancreas** | Trypsin (also activates chymotrypsin) | Proteins, proteoses, peptones, polypeptides | Peptones, peptides, amino acids |
| | Chymotrypsin | Same as trypsin | Same as trypsin |
| | Pancreatic amylase | Starch and dextrins | Dextrins, maltose |
| | Pancreatic lipase | Triglycerides | Fatty acids |
| | Carboxypeptidase | Peptides with a free carboxyl | Glycerol, amino acids |
| **Small Intestine** | Erepsin (a mixture of peptidases) | Peptides, proteoses, peptones | Amino acids |
| | Aminopeptidases | Peptides | Amino acids |
| | Sucrase | Sucrose | Glucose, fructose |
| | Maltase | Maltose | Glucose |
| | Lactase (youngstock) | Lactose | Glucose, galactose |
| | Nucleotidase | Mononucleotides | Nucleosides |
| | Nucleosidase | Nucleosides | Purine and pyrimidine bases, pentoses |
| | Enterokinase | Trypsinogen | Trypsin |

soluble foods will be substantially digested in this relatively short time.

The small intestine also helps to protect the digestive system from infection. It is the only part of the digestive tract with a direct link to the lymphatic system.

# Hindgut

The hindgut acts as a reservoir of water and electrolytes, which is essential for working horses. The rate of feed movement through the hindgut is relatively slow. Because the digestive tract folds back on itself several times and its diameter varies, horses are predisposed to digestive upsets when nutrient flow is abnormal. Since the horse's digestive tract is primarily designed to digest forage, fewer problems occur when the diet is mainly good quality hay or pasture.

# Large intestine

The large intestine comprises the caecum, large colon, small colon and rectum. The large intestine of the horse is approximately 8 m. Although the foregut of the horse is similar to that of other animals with simple stomachs, the hindgut is remarkably different. The large intestine is the site of microbial fermentation and water resorption. There appears to be some compartmentalisation of the large intestine based upon the position of the flexures and sacculations (see Large colon). In these vague compartment areas there is some muscular mixing of ingesta, which is thought to be important for health of the microbial populations required for fermentation of fibre.

The hindgut is where the complex insoluble carbohydrates, cellulose and hemicellulose are digested by fermentation by resident microbial populations.

More than half the dry weight of the horse's faeces is actually microbes. The number of microbes in the digestive tract of the horse is huge, numbering more than ten times the number of cells in the horse's body.

## Caecum

This is a large blind ended, comma shaped sac at the end of the small intestine. The capacity of the caecum is approximately 25–35 l and it is approximately 1.25 m long. Anatomically the caecum has four separate longitudinal bands, which create its characteristic sacculations or pouches.

The caecum acts as a large fermentation vat where fibrous parts of the food are mixed with microorganisms. The flow of digesta into and out of the caecum occurs via a sphincter into the large ventral colon.

## Large colon

The large colon holds approximately 100 l and is 3–4 m long. It consists of four parts namely:

• Right ventral colon (at the base of the caecum)
• Left ventral colon
• Left dorsal colon
• Right dorsal colon.

Anatomically the large colon twists and turns moving backwards into the horse's body and has sharp turns, known as flexures, namely the sternal, pelvic and diaphragmatic flexures. Flexures may be problematical in that blockages may occur at these points causing impactions and colic. The colon also has many bands running across it, similar to the caecum, which create sacculations.

The main function of the caecum and large colon is to house the billions of microbes. These microbial populations are highly susceptible to dietary changes often resulting in digestive upsets such as diarrhoea, colitis, laminitis or colic.

The numbers and species of microbes within the horse's hindgut vary depending upon factors such as ingredients of the diet and any sudden changes to the diet (Table 2.2).

There are many different microbes that are able to break down structural carbohydrates, lactic acid, protein and non-structural carbohydrates that have escaped digestion within the small intestine. These communities thrive within certain areas of the hindgut.

There is a delicate balance between microbes that produce lactic acid and those that convert it to volatile fatty acids (VFAs). Following starch overload, for example, starch will reach the hindgut where it is rapidly broken down by lactobacilli to lactic acid. If bacteria are not present that can reduce the increased lactic acid to VFAs, then the pH will fall and metabolic problems can result (see Chapter 12).

Other functions of the large intestine are:

• Water resorption
• Absorption of B vitamins
• Salt and a small amount of calcium and phosphorus absorption
• Removal of waste/indigestible material.

The small colon is approximately 3.5 m in length and digesta moves from there to the rectum where the faeces are retained until evacuation as droppings.

There are two accessory organs, which carry out functions associated with the digestive system of the horses. These are:

• Pancreas
• Liver.

**Table 2.2** Microbiology of the equine digestive system.

| Site | Protozoa/g ingesta | Total bacteria/g ingesta |
|---|---|---|
| Stomach | 0 | $200 \times 10^6$ |
| Small intestine | 0 | $36 \times 10^6$ |
| Caecum | 567 | $482 \times 10^6$ |
| Large intestine | 567 | $363 \times 10^6$ |

## Pancreas

The pancreas is a gland situated behind the stomach between the spleen and duodenum. It secretes pancreatic juices into the duodenum through a tube known as the pancreatic duct. The cells of the pancreas are divided into insulin and glucagon producing cells of the islets of Langerhans and a network of small alveoli, lined with cells producing digestive enzymes.

The pancreas works with the digestive system and the endocrine (hormone) system. Insulin and glucagon regulate blood sugar levels to maintain a normal range of blood glucose, in the horse.

## Liver

The liver is the largest gland in the horse's body. It is situated immediately behind the diaphragm and in front of the stomach. The horse's liver weighs 5–9 kg. The liver is supplied with blood from two sources; about 75% of this comes via the hepatic portal vein from the stomach and small intestine delivering the products of digestion. The second smaller blood supply to the liver is from the hepatic artery, delivering oxygenated blood from the aorta.

Liver tissue is made up of much smaller units known as liver lobules. These are the site of activity for the many functions of the liver. The liver is vital for cleansing and storage of substances in addition to metabolism.

### Functions of the liver

- The liver removes toxins from harmful substances such as drugs
- Removes nitrogen from amino acids
- Stores glycogen, vitamins A, D, E and K, iron and fats
- Produces heat, vitamins A, D, heparin, plasma proteins (albumin and globulin), prothrombin and fibrinogen, bile, uric acid and urea
- Converts glycogen to glucose, glucose to glycogen, stored fats into other fats such as cholesterol
- Metabolises protein – builds up and breaks down protein
- Produces protein carriers required for transport of fats from the digestive tract.

**Summary points**

- Horses are classed as simple stomached or monogastric.
- Horses like many other animals do not make the enzyme cellulase which is required to break down cellulose.
- The foregut is very similar to that of humans and pigs. The hindgut is similar to the rumen of a cow or a sheep.
- It can take as long as 72 hours for fibrous food to pass through the horse's digestive system.
- Equine teeth differ from human ones in that they slowly erupt continually from the gum throughout the life of the horse.
- Horses have three pairs of salivary glands.
- The stomach is a 'U' shaped elastic organ which is relatively small compared with the overall size of the horse and has a capacity of 10–13 litres.
- The main function of the small intestine is to complete digestion of simple carbohydrates (sugar and starch), lipids (fats and oils), amino acids, vitamins and minerals.
- Horses are not well adapted to digest large amounts of dietary starch.
- The caecum acts as a large fermentation vat where fibrous parts of the food are mixed with microorganisms.
- The main function of the caecum and large colon is to house the billions of microbes that digest fibre producing volatile fatty acids and other products.
- The liver is the largest gland in the horse's body.
- The liver is vital for cleansing and storage of substances in addition to its role in metabolism.

# Food and Biological Molecules

## BIOLOGICAL MOLECULES

A basic knowledge of biological molecules is really important for an understanding of equine nutrition. The sum total of all chemical reactions involving biological molecules in the horse's body is known as metabolism.

All living things are composed of organic compounds containing the chemical elements carbon and hydrogen. Carbon is particularly important because carbon atoms can join together to form long chains or ring structures to which other atoms can attach. In fact it is thought that all life forms evolved from a 'soup' of these organic compounds and that, before life evolved, there was a period of chemical evolution, which resulted in thousands of carbon-based molecules. Methane, ammonia, hydrogen, hydrogen sulphide and water were the building blocks of life itself. At this level chemistry and biology are effectively the same science.

The four groups of biological molecules are:

- Proteins
- Nucleic acids
- Carbohydrates
- Lipids.

These four types of biological molecules compose all life on earth.

Proteins have an enormous variety of functions in all living organisms including the following:

- Biological catalysts
- Forming structural parts of organisms
- Participating in cell signalling and recognition
- Acting as molecules of immunity.

Nucleic acids consist of two distinct but closely related chemical forms:

- Deoxyribonucleic acid (DNA)
- Ribonucleic acid (RNA).

The main functions of these biomolecules include the storage of all genetic and heritable information of all life on earth and the conversion of this information into proteins.

Carbohydrates are the major source of food and the major form of energy for living organisms. When carbohydrates combine together to form long chains or polymers they can also undertake the following functions:

- Long term food storage molecules
- Protective coverings for cells and organisms
- The main structural support for land plants and constituents of many cells and their contents.

Lipids or fats are the major constituents of all membranes in cells. They also serve as food storage molecules.

## Macromolecules

Macromolecules are 'giant' molecules. There are three macromolecules in living organisms:

- Proteins
- Polysaccharides
- Nucleic acids (polynucleotides).

Macromolecules are polymers made up of many similar or identical repeating subunits joined together in long chains:

- Polysaccharides are made up of monosaccharides
- Proteins are made up of amino acids
- Nucleic acids are made up of nucelotides.

## FOOD

The food the horse eats daily is known as the diet. The diet should include the following important nutrients in the correct quantities:

- Water – provides fluid in which other molecules may move
- Carbohydrates – supply energy

- Fats (lipids) – supply energy and help to waterproof the skin
- Protein (amino acids) – building and repair of body tissues and enzymes
- Vitamins required in minute quantities for normal body function
- Minerals (inorganic substances) – for many different life functions

Minerals and vitamins are only required in relatively small amounts.

## Water

The horse's life could not be sustained without water. Approximately 70% of the bodyweight of the horse on a fat free basis is made up of water. Newborn foals may contain as much as 90% water! Water molecules are however very small.

Water is essential for:

- Transport medium
- Temperature regulation
- Medium in which chemical reactions can take place
- Solvent in which substances may be dissolved and transported
- Giving cells their shape
- Excretion in the form of urine
- Milk production.

Essentially all biochemical reactions that occur within the body require water as a vital solvent in which many substances dissolve. Water also acts as a medium for carrying substances in blood, tissue fluids, urine, sweat, and perhaps most importantly within the cytoplasm of cells. Water is the medium of transport around the body including the blood and lymph. Water is also required in many chemical reactions, for example it is used in hydrolysis and results from oxidation reactions.

The most common sources of water for horses are:

- Drinking water
- Free water
- Metabolic water
- Water produced when fat stores are broken down during negative energy balance or starvation (preformed water).

Free water or that contained in a feedstuff releases varying amounts of water. Fresh pasture contains around 75% water (this varies according to stage of growth of the grass). Hay on the other hand has been dried and contains around 10–20% water. A horse consuming 14 kg

(30 lb) fresh pasture will therefore be taking in $14 \times 0.75 = 10.5$ kg water, whereas a horse consuming 7 kg hay will take in $7 \times 0.1 = 0.7$ kg water.

Metabolic water is that derived from oxidation reactions within cells, i.e. metabolic water is bound chemically and released during chemical reactions within the body. The amount of metabolic water produced can be substantial. Some desert animals do not drink water at all as all their needs are matched by metabolic water and the free water contained within food.

The largest amount of water is found within the body tissues as intracellular fluid (i.e. inside cells), particularly muscle cells. Extracellular water (i.e. outside cells) is found in the spaces between cells, plasma, and lymph and within the spinal column and joints. The remaining water is found within the digestive tract and urinary system.

Body water is made up of:

- 40%   Intracellular water
- 33%   Extracellular water
- 27%   Digestive/urinary systems.

## Temperature regulation

Water has excellent properties that make it very useful in temperature regulation. Water has physical properties, which readily enable transfer of heat, build-up of heat and the loss of large amounts of heat through vaporisation. These basic properties act in addition to other physiological factors such as the circulation of large volumes of blood (fluid), large surface areas for evaporation on the skin and within the lungs. Horses are able to divert blood to the body surfaces for sweating when the horse is getting too warm and also divert blood away from the body surface in cold ambient temperatures.

Loss of too much water from the horse's body will cause dehydration and eventually death and therefore it is important for the body to readily absorb water from the digestive tract and maintain fluid balance by absorbing water via the kidneys when required. Water is lost from the horse's body via urine, faeces, sweat and evaporation from the lungs and skin. Withholding water has dangerous implications causing dehydration and colic. Loss of too much water from the digestive tract such as in diarrhoea can be life threatening, particularly for young foals. Losses of 5–10% of bodyweight have been found in competing endurance horses. Voluntary water intake by horses at rest in a moderate temperature environment is roughly 25–70 ml/kg/day. For a 500 kg horse this equates to 12.5–35 litres per day. This depends on the balance between water intake from the feed and drinking and water losses.

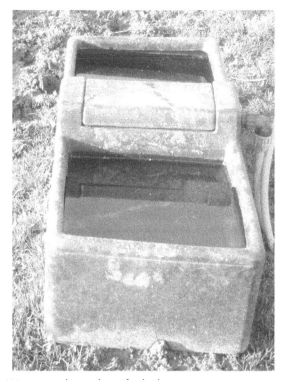

**Figure 3.1**   Water trough supplying fresh clean water.

If horses are given too much protein, i.e. in excess of requirements, more water will be required as excess protein must be broken down and the excess nitrogen removed via the urine. Increased salt intake also increases water intake. A supply of fresh clean water is vital for all horses (Figure 3.1).

## Carbohydrates

Carbohydrates are the main component of all plants including those which horses eat. They make up roughly 70% of the dry matter (dry matter is the material left when the food has been dried and all water removed).

The name carbohydrate is derived from the French term *hydrate de carbone*. Carbohydrates are made up of the elements carbon (C), hydrogen (H) and oxygen (O) often referred to as CHOs. Carbohydrates include starch, glycogen and cellulose and many other compounds; cereal grains may contain as much as 85% carbohydrate in the dry matter.

Most importantly carbohydrates are the most common constituent in horse feeds (after water has been removed), making up roughly 80%

of the dry matter of cereal grains and 70% of the dry matter of forage. Carbohydrates are made within the leaves of all living green plants, by the process of photosynthesis (Chapter 2).

Less than 1% of the weight of a horse is made up of the carbohydrate glucose and its storage form, glycogen. Dietary carbohydrate is the main energy source for horses and includes starches and sugars. Glycogen is the storage form of glucose in all mammals. Some of the important carbohydrates for horses are shown in Table 3.1.

Carbohydrates may be termed as simple or complex, structural (SC) or non-structural (NSC), water soluble (WSC), or non-starch.

Major sources of carbohydrates in equine nutrition are shown in Figure 3.2.

In their most basic form carbohydrates are monosaccharides or simple sugars, which can combine with each other to form more complex carbohydrates:

- Disaccharide – combination of 2 simple sugars
- Oligosaccharide – combination of 2–10 simple sugars
- Polysaccharide – more than 10 simple sugars.

**Table 3.1**  Examples of carbohydrates.

|  | Monosaccharide contained in: | Found naturally in: |
|---|---|---|
| ***Monosaccharide (simple sugar)*** | | |
| *Pentose* | N/A | Corn cobs |
| Xylose | | |
| *Hexose* | N/A | |
| Glucose | | |
| ***Disaccharide (complex)*** | | |
| *Sucrose* | Glucose-fructose | Sugar beet, sugar cane, table sugar |
| Maltose | Glucose-glucose | Starchy plants, roots |
| Lactose | Glucose-galactose | Milk |
| ***Polysaccharide (complex)*** | | |
| *Pentosans* | | |
| Araban | Arabinose | Pectins |
| *Hexosans* | | |
| Starch | Glucose | Cereal grain, seeds and tubers |
| Cellulose | Glucose | Plant cell walls |
| Glycogen | Glucose | Muscle and liver cells of horses |
| ***Mixed polysaccharides*** | | |
| Hemicellulose | Mixtures of pentoses and hexoses | Plant fibre |

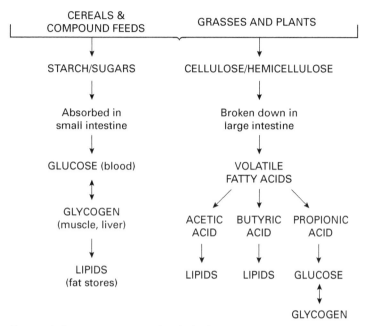

**Figure 3.2**  Major sources of carbohydrates in equine nutrition.

Each disaccharide contains one unit of glucose and glucose is the unit from which all polysaccharides are made. These four types of carbohydrates are interchangeable in that monosaccharides may be built up into disaccharides and polysaccharides. Polysaccharides may be broken down into disaccharides and monosaccharides. There are far more disaccharides and polysaccharides in plants than monosaccharides.

Sugars are also known as soluble carbohydrates and polysaccharides as insoluble carbohydrates.

## Monosaccharides

These are simple sugars that dissolve easily in water to form a sweet tasting solution and are classified by the number of carbon atoms they contain:

- 4 (Tetrose) – e.g. erythrose, threose
- 5 (Pentose) – e.g. arabinose, ribose, ribulose, xylose, xylulose
- 6 (Hexose) –e.g. allose, fructose, galactose, glucose, idose, mannose, sorbose, talose
- 7 (Heptose) – e.g. sedoheptulose.

The names of all sugars end in 'ose'. Many structures differ only very slightly and this depends upon the orientation of the OH or hydroxyl group. The very slight difference in structure produces very different biochemical properties, taste being one of them. Hexose sugars including glucose and fructose have the molecular formula $C_6H_{12}O_6$. (Figure 3.3).

The main monosaccharides are glucose, fructose, galactose, mannose, arabinose and xylose. These monosaccharides are found in low concentrations in plants but are found in some oligosaccharides and polysaccharides in horse feeds. These are the building blocks of the naturally occurring disaccharides, oligosaccharides and polysaccharides. Free glucose and fructose can be found in honey and in small amounts in carrots. Monosaccharides play extremely important roles within the horse's body. Firstly they have the ability to move across living membranes between and within all living cells. Only monosaccharides can pass through the wall of the small intestine hence larger carbohydrates must be broken down by digestion to these small units before absorption. Monosaccharides provide a source of carbohydrate and therefore energy for all living cells. Monosaccharides create the first and vital stage of release of chemical energy from a long chain of reactions. Because monosaccharides are relatively small and soluble in water, they are the form in which carbohydrates are carried round the body in the bloodstream.

The simplest carbohydrates are the simple sugars such as glucose and fructose. These are single unit sugars from the Greek *mono* (single) and *sacchar* (sugar). Glucose is the main fuel for all cells and is the sugar commonly known as 'blood sugar'. Glucose is perhaps the most well known carbohydrate and its molecular formula is ($C_6H_{12}O_6$).

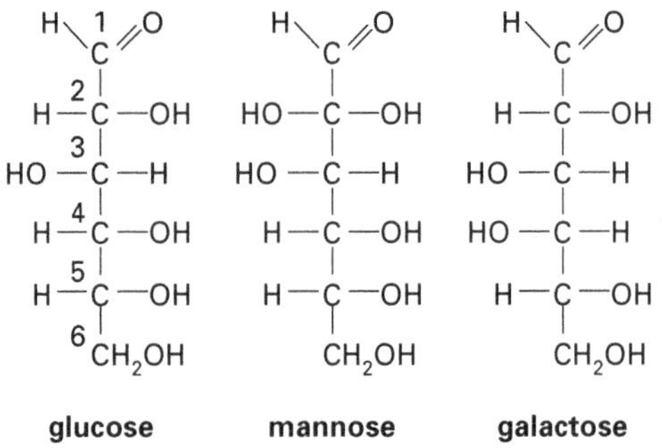

**Figure 3.3** Example of a monosaccharide, e.g. glucose.

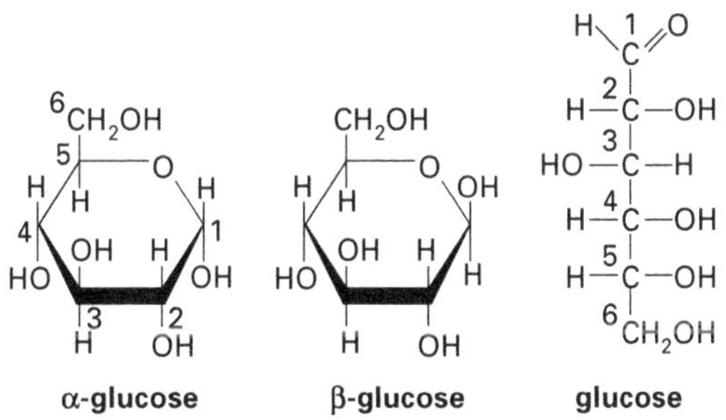

**Figure 3.4**   Structure of glucose.

Pentose and hexose sugars can exist in a chain or the more stable ring form as the chain of carbons is long enough to close up on itself. When glucose forms a ring, the first carbon atom joins to the oxygen atom on the fifth carbon atom. The structure of the glucose molecule is a six-sided ring (hence the term hexose sugar) (Figure 3.4). The hydroxyl or OH group may be situated above or below the carbon ring in glucose. If below, it is known as alpha-glucose and if above beta-glucose. These are two forms of the same chemical and are known as isomers and have important consequences in the structures of glycogen, starch and cellulose.

Fructose is also referred to as fruit sugar; this sugar is the sweetest of sugars and is the one that makes fruit and honey taste sweet. Fructose has the same chemical formula as glucose but is different in structure.

Galactose is also a monosaccharide occurring rarely in its free state in nature. It combines with glucose to form lactose (a disaccharide) i.e. milk sugar (see below).

Monosaccharides have very important roles in the horse'sbody:

• As a source of energy for respiration in cells including muscle cells – due to the high number of carbon–hydrogen bonds which can be broken to release large amounts of energy to make ATP (adenosine triphosphate) (see Chapter 6)
• As building blocks for much larger molecules such as starch, glycogen and cellulose. Glucose, for example, is used to make the polysaccharides glycogen, starch and cellulose.

### Disaccharides

Disaccharides consist of two glucose or similar monosaccharides joined together (Figure 3.5).

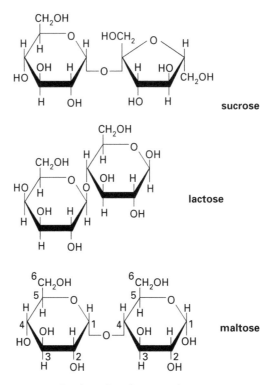

**Figure 3.5**  Structure of a disaccharide (examples).

## Sucrose

Sucrose is more commonly known as ordinary table sugar refined from sugar beet or sugar cane. Sucrose is one glucose molecule joined to one fructose molecule. The molecular formula of sucrose is $C_{12}H_{22}O_{11}$.

## Lactose

Lactose or milk sugar is another disaccharide; it is formed from glucose and galactose. Young foals use the enzyme lactase to break down lactose in the small intestine.

## Maltose

Maltose consists of two alpha glucose molecules joined together by a link termed a glycosidic link or bond. Maltose is roughly 30% as sweet as sucrose or table sugar. Maltose is a disaccharide made from two glucose molecules and is produced when starch is broken down during digestion. It is a disaccharide derived from starch and is found in sprouted wheat and barley.

## Glycosidic bond

Two monosaccharides may be joined together by a bridge known as the glycosidic bond. This basically means that the hydroxyl (OH) group from each of two monosaccharides combine to form water, which is removed leaving an oxygen bridge in the resulting disaccharide (Figure 3.6). This reaction is known as condensation. The reverse can happen whereby water is added to a disaccharide by a process known as hydrolysis to break it down to form two monosaccharides. The link is important as it enables the rapid build up and break down of important molecules such as glycogen within the body.

## Short chain carbohydrates or oligosaccharides

Better known as short chain carbohydrates, they are composed of chains of 3–10 monosaccharide units. Oligosaccharides in food fall into two groups: the maltodextrins that are mainly derived from starch and the others such as raffinose (a trisaccharide), stachyose and verbascose. These are effectively sucrose joined to varying numbers of galactose molecules and are found in beans and peas.

## Fructo-oligosaccharides

Also within this group are the fructo-oligosaccharides (FOS) and inulin. These are fructans and are storage carbohydrates found in herbage. Fructan is often used to describe molecules containing many fructose units and so both inulin and FOS are types of fructans. Some plants store carbohydrate as inulin in addition to or instead of starch. Inulin is found in garlic and in many vegetables. Inulins are

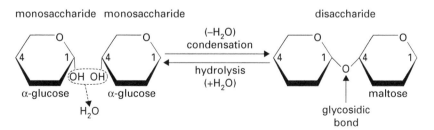

**Figure 3.6**  Glycosidic bond making a disaccharide.

polymers consisting of many units of fructose with most typically glucose at the end of the chain. Oligofructose has the same structure but the chains are smaller in number than inulin consisting of 10 or fewer units of fructose. Oligofructose and inulin cannot be digested in the small intestine of the horse by enzymic digestion and are therefore fermented by hindgut microbes producing volatile fatty acids and lactate.

Some short chain carbohydrates are used to stimulate the growth of beneficial microbes in the hindgut and these are better known as preprobiotics (see Chapter 9).

## Polysaccharides – complex carbohydrates

These are long chains of sugar molecules from a few hundred to several thousand units. They are classified as starch and non-starch polysaccharides. Many polysaccharides are insoluble in water, unlike sugars. Essentially the fibre part of the diet for horses includes polysaccharides that are resistant to digestion in the equine small intestine but are fermented in the hindgut by the microbial population that live there.

## Starch

Starch is the storage polysaccharide of plants such as cereals and root vegetables including carrots. Starch consists of long chains of glucose molecules and is found in plants in partially crystalline form and within plant cells as starch granules. Cereal grains are major sources of starch, supplying a concentrated form of energy. Starch consists of two types of polysaccharide namely:

- Amylose – long unbranched chain of glucose molecules
- Amylopectin – large, highly branched chain of glucose molecules.

Most cereal starches contain 15–30% amylose. Some more waxy starches contain higher amounts of amylopectin and these include the starch found in barley and maize. This is the major form of stored carbohydrate in all plants and consists of amylose and amylopectin. Starch is never found in animal cells. Amylose is essentially linear in structure while amylopectin is highly branched, but both consist of chains of alpha glucose. Amylose (Figure 3.7) consits of 200 to 20,000 units of glucose which form a helix.

Amylopectin (Figure 3.7) is highly branched with short side chains of about 30 glucose units and may contain as many as two million glucose units. Hydrolysis uses water and enzymes to break down the

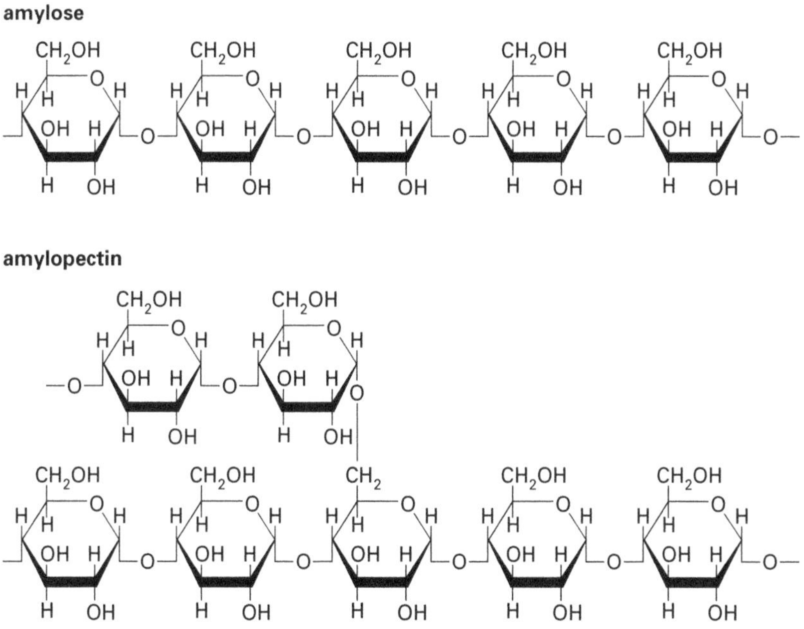

amylose

amylopectin

**Figure 3.7**  Amylose and amylopectin structure.

long starch chains into smaller units or simple carbohydrates (see above).

All starch is potentially digested by α-amylase in the digestive tract, however it is not always digested at the same rate, as some starches are more resistant to this enzymic digestion. Cooking, micronising and extruding all help to make starch in cereal grains more digestible and therefore available to the horse.

## Glycogen

Glycogen is another storage polysaccharide, with a structure identical to amylopectin but the branches in glycogen are shorter. It is made up of long chains of alpha-glucose molecules. Glycogen is the body's form of stored carbohydrate and is easily converted back to glucose for energy. Both starch and glycogen may be broken down into their constituent glucose units by breakage of the links joining them together. Horses have enzymes to break down these links.

## Non-starch polysaccharides (NSP)/structural carbohydrates

Non-starch polysaccharides or structural carbohydrates are essentially the polysaccharides of the plant cell wall. Cellulose consists of long

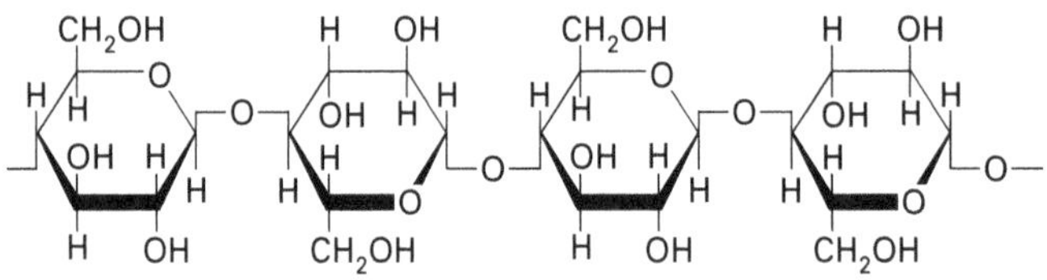

**Figure 3.8**   Structure of cellulose.

unbranched linear chains. Cellulose is made up of chains of beta-glucose whereas starch and glycogen are made up of chains of alpha-glucose (Figure 3.8).

The absence of side chains allows cellulose molecules to lie close together and form rigid structures. Cellulose is therefore the major structural material of plants and provides the rigid structure required to hold plants upright. Cellulose fibres have very strong tensile strength, indeed almost as strong as steel and therefore help give plants their structure. Cellulose is the most abundant organic substance found in nature and so it provides a great supply of carbohydrate if the links holding the chain together can be broken. Ruminants and hindgut fermentors such as the horse have found a way to break these links through microbial fermentation (see below).

The beta-glucose units (up to 10,000) of cellulose have different links from those in starch. The glucose links in cellulose cannot be broken down by the horse's own digestive enzymes. The horse, like all herbivores, needs microbes, which produce the enzyme cellulase to break down cellulose (see Chapter 1).

The hemicelluloses are a diverse group of NSPs that contain a mixture of pentose (5C) and hexose (6C) sugars in long, often highly branched chains which are shorter than cellulose at around 50–2000 units. Hemicelluloses comprise almost one third of the carbohydrates in woody plant tissue. Hemicelluloses may be found in plant stems and grain hulls. Although hemicelluloses are not digestible, they can be fermented by microbes in the hindgut. A typical hemicellulose is arabinoxylans found in cereals. Other soluble NSPs include pectins and gums.

The carbohydrate available to the horse in green plants is largely provided by:

- Cell contents – simple sugars and starches that are digested in the small intestine
- Cell walls – cellulose/ hemicellulose fermented by micro-organisms in the hindgut to VFAs (volatile fatty acids).

## Volatile fatty acids (VFAs)

Most if not all the non-structural carbohydrate that enters the hindgut of the horse will be fermented resulting in volatile fatty acids. This excludes that associated with lignin, which reduces fermentation of NSPs. VFAs are produced in large quantities by microbial fermentation within the caecum and to a lesser extent in the colon of the horse. This is an anaerobic process and the resulting VFAs are then absorbed through the caecal and colonic epithelium or lining, before being distributed around the horse's body for use as energy sources.

In the horse the majority of energy supplied to the body is derived from microbial digestion of both plant fibre and soluble carbohydrate. Anaerobic fermentation of starch and cellulose produces large quantities of VFAs, namely:

- Acetic acid – short chain
- Butyric acid – short chain
- Propionic acid – short chain
- Isobutyric acid
- Valeric acid and isovaleric acid

Additional products include lactic acid, $CO_2$ and methane.

The most important VFAs are propionate, butyrate and acetate. These are collected via the hepatic portal system and transferred to the liver. Propionate is then converted to glucose in the liver. Acetate and butyrate are used for fat synthesis and also as an aerobic energy supply.

VFAs therefore contribute a substantial amount of energy to the horse.

## Carbohydrate metabolism

Blood glucose in horses rises following feeds high in cereal starch such as coarse mixes or straights. Insulin is then released from the pancreas, which results in the uptake of glucose by cells including muscle and fat cells (see Chapter 7). Absorbed glucose is either used for energy or stored as glycogen or fat for later use. Glycogen is stored in the muscle cells and liver. This is explained in Chapter 5.

## Protein

Protein is a constituent of every cell and tissue within the horse's body, including muscle, skin, tendons, hair and hooves. Protein makes up about 18% of the horse's body. All cells within the horse's body produce thousands of different proteins. More than 50% of the dry mass of all living cells is made up of protein. Protein is required for:

- Growth and formation of new tissues
- Repair and renewal of old tissues
- Synthesis of most hormones and enzymes and neurotransmitters
- Maintaining fluid balance within tissues
- Regulation of blood clotting
- Antibodies
- Collagen – adds strength to many tissues including bone
- Haemoglobin in red blood cells
- Transport of substances in and out of cells
- Hair and skin which contain the protein keratin.

Proteins are organic molecules, which not only contain carbon, hydrogen, and oxygen (similar to carbohydrates) but also contain nitrogen and small amounts of sulphur.

All body cells make proteins and without proteins life would not exist. Similar to polysaccharides, proteins are made up of long chains of smaller units called amino acids joined end to end. Proteins or amino acids must be provided in the horse's diet to enable normal growth and life processes. Twenty individual amino acids, which are the building blocks of proteins, may be joined together in chains in different sequences to make individual proteins. Each individual protein has its own unique chain of amino acids in a specific order for that protein and there are millions of different proteins. A protein molecule may contain hundreds or thousands of amino acids units in the chain and each link between two amino acids is known as a peptide link.

**Table 3.2** Essential and non-essential amino acids.

| Essential amino acids | Non-essential amino acids |
| --- | --- |
| Isoleucine | Alanine |
| Leucine | Asparagine |
| Lysine | Cysteine |
| Methionine | Glutamic acid |
| Phenylalanine | Glutamine |
| Threonine | Glycine |
| Tryptophan | Proline |
| Valine | Serine |
| Arginine | Tyrosine |
| Histidine – essential for foals | Aspartate |

Horses are able to make some amino acids themselves within the body from other amino acids, nitrogen and carbohydrate. These are known as *non-essential* or *dispensable*. Others must be supplied in the diet and are known as *essential* or *indispensable* amino acids (see Table 3.2).

## Protein structure

The general structure for all amino acids is shown in Figure 3.9. All have a central carbon atom to which is bonded an amine group ($NH_2$) and a carboxylic group (COOH). The third component bonded to a carbon atom is always hydrogen. R varies according to the individual protein and is known as the R group or side chain. In other words only the R group differs in individual amino acids.

### Peptide bond

Amino acids may be joined together by a condensation reaction, i.e. water is removed. This is similar to the formation of a glycosidic bond in disaccharides and in the synthesis of fats. The new molecule consists of two amino acid units and is known as a dipeptide. Many more amino acid units can be added by this condensation reaction to form polypeptides. Polypeptides and dipeptides can also be broken down by the addition of water or hydrolysis, again similar to the breaking of the glycosidic bond to produce smaller chains of amino acids or amino acids This occurs in the stomach and small intestine during digestion of protein molecules in the horse's food. Polypeptides are macromolecules.

The structure of proteins may be referred to in several ways:

1. Primary structure – the unique sequence of amino acids in the chain
2. Secondary structure – coils and folds of the protein of which there are two types

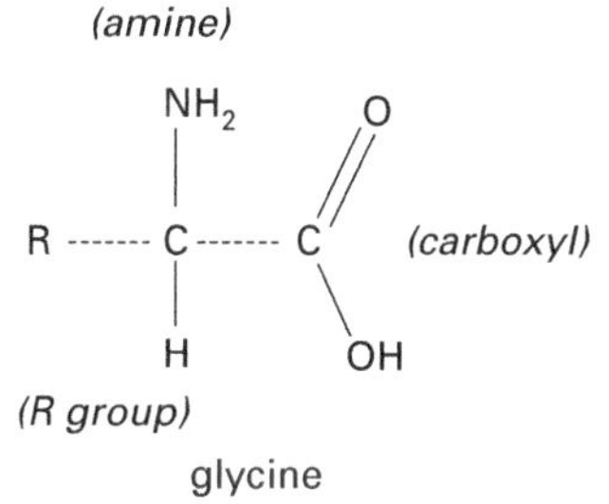

**Figure 3.9**  General structure of an amino acid.

   a) alpha helix delicate coil
   b) beta pleated sheet
3. Tertiary structure: superimposed patterns of secondary structure
4. Quaternary structure: association of different polypeptide chains, e.g. haemoglobin.

The molecules in some proteins curl up into a ball structure and these are called globular proteins. Some amino acids have a branched configuration and are known as branched chain amino acids (BCAAs). Three essential amino acids with this branched shape are valine, leucine and isoleucine. They make up approximately one third of muscle protein.

Proteins vary tremendously in composition, properties, size, shape and function. Some proteins are soluble, such as haemoglobin found in red blood cells, others are insoluble, such as keratin found in hooves and mane and tail hair.

There are many reactions going on simultaneously in cells. Enzymes enable these reactions to take place quickly at body temperature. All enzymes are proteins and this helps demonstrate the importance of proteins in the physiology of the horse. Proteins are also used to make antibodies to help horses fight disease. Growing foals and pregnant and lactating mares need high quality protein which supplies higher numbers of essential amino acids to support growth.

Unlike carbohydrates, proteins are not a major energy source, only when the horse is in a negative energy balance or starvation will body tissues be broken down releasing protein as a last resort to produce energy.

## Lipids (fats)

Lipids are concentrated sources of energy. Lipids are a diverse group of chemical compounds, the most common of which are the triglycerides which are more usually known as fats and oils. Fats are solid at room temperature whereas oils are liquid. Fat acts as en energy store and 1 g of fat gives about 39 kJ of energy more than twice as much as that released by 1 g of carbohydrate (see Chapter 4). Body fats within the horse are rapidly mobilised during exercise.

Each triglyceride is made up of one molecule of glycerol and three fatty acids attached to it (Figure 3.10). The fatty acid is joined with the glycerol molecule by the loss of water or a condensation reaction. Each fatty acid consists of a chain of carbon atoms (with hydrogen atoms attached) of different lengths usually between 14 and 22 carbons with

glycerol + 3 fatty acids                                    triglyceride molecule

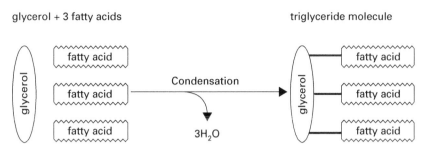

**Figure 3.10**   Structure of a triglyceride.

a carboxyl group (–COOH) and a methyl group (–CH3) at either end. Fatty acids are classified according to their chemical structure:

• Saturated
• Monounsaturated
• Polyunsaturated.

Lipids make excellent energy sources and storage compounds in the horse's body because they are even richer in carbon–hydrogen bonds than carbohydrates.

## Essential fatty acids

Some polyunsaturated fats cannot be made by the horse's body and must be supplied in the diet, they are known as *essential* fatty acids. There are two essential fatty acids that all horses need in the diet, namely omega-3 and omega-6. Important essential omega-3 fatty acids are α-linolenic acid (ALA), eicosapentaenoic acid (EPA), and docosahexaenoic acid (DHA).

A relationship exists between the types and amount of fats and health, inflammation and development. A balance of these is required as there is competition within these two 'fat' families within the body. Both omega-3 and omega-6 fatty acids have very different metabolic pathways.

Omega-6 (Linoleic acid) → Gamma Linolenic (GLA) → Arachidonic acid
Omega-3 (Linolenic acid)(**ALA**) → Eicosapentaenoic acid (**EPA**) →
    Docosahexaenoic acid (**DHA**)

Of these DHA and EPA are particularly vital and have important roles providing protection against degenerative disease and illness. DHA and EPA are thought to reduce inflammation and thereby assist in joint and respiratory function and also aid fertility in the mare and stallion.

Horses with 24 hour access to good quality pasture can obtain these essential fatty acids in the correct balance. However, quality of pasture varies throughout the year. Flaxseed or linseed oil and fish oil are the most well known sources of omega-3s but only a small percentage of omega-3 from flaxseed oil gets converted to the important EPA or DHA, about 3%. Fish oil however converts about 30%, ten times more. Not all fish oils contain high levels of omega-3 fatty acids. Fish from warm tropical waters have a diet of plankton rich in EPA and DHA. Fish from within warm tropical waters therefore are the richest source of EPA and DHA. EPA and DHA are important ingredients of the horse's diet.

Feeding EPA and DHA will help redress the balance when cereal-based feeds are fed and where pasture is at all limited, helping to encourage anti-inflammatory pathways and improve autoimmune function. Breeding stock may receive additional benefits such as improved colostrum quality, sperm quality and correct development of the foetus.

---

**Summary points**

- The four groups of biological molecules are proteins, nucleic acids carbohydrates and lipids.
- Carbohydrates are the major source of food and the major form of energy for living organisms.
- Macromolecules are 'giant' molecules – there are three macromolecules in living organisms namely proteins, polysaccharides and nucleic acids (polynucleotides).
- Carbohydrates are the most common constituent in horse feeds.
- Carbohydrates are made up of the elements carbon (C), hydrogen (H) and oxygen (O) often referred to as CHOs.
- In their most basic form carbohydrates are monosaccharides or simple sugars, which can combine with each other to form more complex carbohydrates.
- Monosaccharides provide a source of carbohydrate and therefore energy for all living cells.
- Some short chain carbohydrates are used to stimulate the growth of the healthy bacteria in the hindgut and these are better known as preprobiotics.
- Starch is the major form of stored carbohydrate in all plants and consists of amylose and amylopectin.
- Starch and glycogen are polymers of alpha-glucose whereas cellulose is a polmer of beta-glucose.
- Cellulose is the most abundant organic substance found in nature and provides an abundant supply of carbohydrate if the links holding the chain together can be broken.

- The main products of fermentation of fibre are the short chain VFAs, propionate, butyrate and acetate.
- Additional products of fermentation are lactic acid, $CO_2$ and methane.
- Protein is a constituent of every cell and tissue within the horse's body, including muscle, skin, tendons, hair and hooves.
- More than 50% of the dry mass of all living cells is made up of protein.
- Proteins vary tremendously in composition, properties, size, shape and function.
- Growing foals and pregnant/lactating mares need high quality protein which supplies higher numbers of essential amino acids to support growth.
- Proteins are not a major energy source.
- Lipids are concentrated sources of energy that can be quickly used by the horse.
- Lipids are a diverse group of chemical compounds, the most common of which are the triglycerides usually known as fats and oils.
- Some polyunsaturated fats cannot be made by the horse's body and so must be supplied in the diet, they are known as *essential* fatty acids – omega-3 and omega-6 fatty acids

# Vitamins

Vitamins are required in minute quantities for optimum health, hence they are known as micronutrients. Working, breeding and lactating horses depend upon a balance of these important nutrients for peak growth and performance. The horse's body relies upon millions of chemical reactions taking place within the cells. Many of these reactions require substances to speed the reactions up, namely catalysts and these are enzymes (proteins). Catalysts often need additional cofactors such as minerals or organic vitamins to work properly.

Vitamins are organic compounds that are either supplied in the horse's diet or the horse can make them within the body, mostly within the hindgut. Unlike humans, horses can mostly synthesise their own vitamins apart from vitamins A and E. Vitamins play essential roles within enzyme systems involved in metabolism. They are required as cofactors for enzymes involved in many cellular reactions including the energy production process and within the immune, nervous and hormonal systems. Even so, vitamins are only required in tiny amounts (milligrams or in some cases micrograms). Excessive quantities of vitamins can also be dangerous, depending upon the vitamin concerned. The horse's body can store some vitamins, but not others. Nutrient Requirements of Horses (NRC 2007) has estimated requirements for vitamins A, D and E, thiamine and riboflavin, however there is as yet insufficient information available to provide accurate requirements for the other vitamins for horses.

Vitamins are often unstable and therefore easily destroyed. If vitamins are not supplied to the body, horses will become deficient and the body cells will begin to fail, ultimately leading to death.

Vitamins and their functions and sources are shown in Table 4.1.

**Table 4.1** Functions, sources and deficiencies of vitamins in horses.

| Vitamin | Required for | Source | Deficiency signs |
|---|---|---|---|
| | FAT | SOLUBLE | VITAMINS |
| A<br>Carotenoids, e.g<br>  beta-carotene or<br>  is converted to<br>  retinol | Healthy eyes<br>Immune system<br>Growth &<br>  maintenance<br>  of body tissues | Grass<br>Green forage | Lack of appetite<br>Night blindness<br>Poor growth<br>Keratinisation of eyes<br>Hoof and skin in poor<br>  condition<br>Infertility |
| D<br>Sunshine vitamin | Aids absorption<br>  of calcium and<br>  phosphorus in<br>  the gut<br>Bone formation<br>Joint integrity | Horses synthesise<br>  Vitamin D in their<br>  skin in the pres-<br>  ence of sunlight.<br>Sun dried hay<br>  (stabled horses<br>  may need<br>  supplementing) | Bones fail to calcify<br>  leading to rickets in<br>  young horses and<br>  osteomalacia in<br>  older ones<br>Swollen joints<br>Fractures |
| E<br>Tocopherols | Muscle integrity<br>Fat metabolism<br>Acts with sele-<br>  nium as an<br>  antioxidant<br>Reproduction | Alfalfa<br>Green forage<br>Cereals | Muscular disorders<br>Infertility |
| K | Blood clotting | Produced by healthy<br>  hindgut microbial<br>  population<br>Leafy forage | True deficiency is<br>  rare<br>Levels can be<br>  assessed by<br>  measuring blood<br>  clotting time |
| | WATER | SOLUBLE | VITAMINS |
| C<br>Ascorbic acid | Immune system<br>Antioxidant<br>Muscle and<br>  blood capillary<br>  integrity | Made in body tissues<br>  from glucose | Bleeding, ulcerated<br>  gums.<br>Internal bleeding<br>Interacts with copper<br>  and iron. |
| $B_1$<br>Thiamine | Fat and carbohy-<br>  drate<br>  metabolism,<br>  particularly<br>  glucose | Produced by healthy<br>  hind gut microbial<br>  population | Deficiency may be<br>  caused by eating<br>  bracken<br>Loss of appetite<br>Incoordination<br>Staggering |
| $B_2$<br>Riboflavin | Carbohydrate,<br>  protein and fat<br>  metabolism | Produced by healthy<br>  hindgut microbial<br>  population | Reduced growth rate<br>Reduced utilisation<br>  of feed<br>Possibly involved in<br>  periodic ophthalmia |
| $B_6$<br>Pyridoxine<br>  was known as<br>  Vit H | Carbohydrate,<br>  protein and fat<br>  metabolism<br>Enzyme systems | Grass<br>Green forage | In absence of $B_6$,<br>  tryptophan and<br>  niacin<br>cannot be utilised<br>Poor growth,<br>  dermatitis<br>Nerve degeneration |

**Table 4.1**  *Continued*

| Vitamin | Required for | Source | Deficiency signs |
|---|---|---|---|
| | *WATER* | *SOLUBLE* | *VITAMINS* |
| $B_{12}$ Cyanocobalamin | Carbohydrate, fat and protein metabolism | Produced by healthy hindgut microbial population, but requires cobalt to do this | Poor growth Infertility Poor appetite Rough coat |
| Folic acid Folacin | Maturation of red blood cells Interacts with $B_2$, $B_{12}$,C | Grass Green forage Synthesised in hindgut by healthy microbial population | Not described in horses |
| Biotin | Hoof horn production Carbohydrate protein and fat metabolism | Maize, yeast, soya Green forage | Poor hoof condition, hoof crumbles at ground surface |
| Niacin Nicotinic acid | Enzyme systems in all body cells. Cell integrity and metabolism Carbohydrate, protein and fat digestion | Can be synthesised from the amino acid tryptophan Cereals | Never been produced in the horse |
| Pantothenic acid Calcium pantothenate | Part of co-enzymes Carbohydrate, fat and protein digestion | Synthesised in hindgut by healthy microbial population | No specific deficiency signs seen in horses. |

Vitamins are grouped according to their solubility in fat or water into two broad categories namely:

- Fat soluble
- Water soluble.

## FAT SOLUBLE VITAMINS

Fat soluble vitamins include vitamins A, D, E and K. This group depends upon fat for absorption and transport from the digestive tract and any excess is stored in the horse's fat stores. They are insoluble in water and so cannot be excreted in the urine if excess to requirements, instead they accumulate in the liver and fat stores where they may become harmful.

Fat soluble vitamins require fat or lipid carriers to transport them around the body. Vitamins A and E are not actually made within the horse's body and therefore must be supplied in the diet. Green forages, however, are rich sources of these two important vitamins.

## Vitamin A/carotenoids

Vitamin A is otherwise known as retinol or retinoic acid. All green plants contains a class of pigments known as carotenoids of which the most important is beta-carotene, which horses can then convert to vitamin A in the body. These carotenoids are generically known as provitamin A and there are roughly 500 of them with vitamin A activity. In fact, 1 µg beta-carotene is equivalent to 400 IU vitamin A.

Although the conversion of carotenoids to retinol is not very inefficient, most horses consume great quantities of green forage and deficiency is therefore rare. Beta-carotene is broken down to retinol prior to absorption across the intestinal membrane in the horse's digestive tract. Once absorbed it is incorporated into small structures known as chylomicrons for transport around the body. Beta-carotene is a powerful antioxidant that helps to destroy free radicals that are normally produced during metabolism but they can damage healthy cells and so must be effectively 'mopped up' by antioxidants. Beta-carotene also enhances vitamin E's antioxidant function, by aiding regeneration.

Vitamin A is required for:

- Night vision
- Epithelial cells (lining cells such as the lining of the gut, respiratory tract, genitourinary tract, respiratory tract and skin)
- Bone growth and remodelling
- Important antioxidant activities
- Wound healing
- Boosting the immune system.

The daily requirement of vitamin A for a 500 kg horse is given by NRC 2007 as 15,000 IU for horses at maintenance, 22,500 IU for horses in work and 30,000 IU for pregnant and lactating mares.

Vitamin A deficiency is very unlikely in horses at pasture. Green forage is rich in vitamin A and grazing horses are able to store excess vitamin A in the liver providing a supply for 3–6 months when pasture is in short supply such as over the winter months. Breeding mares, particularly thoroughbreds preparing for early breeding may benefit from beta-carotene supplementation through the winter. Horses fed recommended amounts of compound feeds should receive adequate amounts of vitamins and are therefore unlikely to be deficient.

However, owing to poor nutritional management and/or poor health, some horses may show deficiency symptoms such as:

- Night blindness
- Slow growth rate
- Infertility
- Dull coat
- Anorexia and weight loss
- Infections
- Enteritis.

Horses on diets that provide less than 500 IU vitamin A/kg DM (dry matter) or those receiving little green forage are more likely to become deficient and show symptoms. Although vitamin A is a powerful antioxidant it also plays a vital role in maintaining immunity and strengthening resistance, important factors for working and breeding horses.

Because carotenes are gradually destroyed by heat and light, beta-carotene in hay is lost fairly rapidly and after six months' storage there is little if any left. The traditional practice of feeding hay over one year old is therefore not recommended. However, dehydrated forages such as dried alfalfa and grass that has been rapidly dried under high temperatures retain much of their beta-carotene.

As a general rule the greener the forage the more carotene it contains.

Excess vitamin A is not excreted easily and so high intakes over long periods may result in toxicity symptoms. Feeding greater than 20,000 IU vitamin A/kg of diet per day may induce toxicity and signs including anorexia, weight loss, thickening and scaling of skin, dull coat, anaemia, reduced bone strength and reduced kidney and liver function.

## Vitamin D

Vitamin D is known as the sunshine vitamin. It is found in higher concentrations in cut dried forages than in fresh pasture. Horses are able to synthesise another form of vitamin D, vitamin D3 or cholecalciferol from a provitamin, which is formed within the horse's skin in the presence of UV light. In the United Kingdom, for example, little or no vitamin D synthesis occurs in the skin from October to March because of lack of the correct wavelength of light. Consequently, vitamin D made during the summer months in excess of requirements will be stored within the horse's body for use over the winter months.

Horses stabled all year round are likely to need dietary sources of vitamin D, as they are unable to synthesise their own. It is important for horses out in the spring and summer to be kept without rugs to enable the skin to make sufficient vitamin D. Fat soluble vitamins, including both ingested and skin manufactured vitamin D, are transported in chylomicrons within the lymphatic system firstly to the liver and then to the kidneys where vitamin D is converted via further reactions to its most active form namely calcitrol. Vitamin D is vital for calcium and phosphorus metabolism. The main function of vitamin D is to maintain levels of calcium and phosphorus within the horse's blood at an appropriate level for bone growth and remodelling, proper functioning of nerve and muscle tissue and support of metabolism within cells. Vitamin D is also essential for blood clotting.

When plasma calcium levels drop too low, a hormone known as parathyroid hormone is released which stimulates the production of calcitrol within the horse's kidneys. This results in more dietary calcium being absorbed in the intestine, a reduction in calcium loss from the kidneys and an increase in calcium mobilisation from bone. All these result in increased plasma calcium. It is important to note however that vitamin D will not compensate for persistently low levels of dietary calcium and/or phosphorus. Horses that are out in sunlight for several hours daily or that are fed sun-dried hay in significant quantities are unlikely to be deficient in vitamin D. However, permanently stabled horses on low forage rations will need vitamin D supplementation.

The daily requirement for a 500 kg horse is 3300 IU/day of vitamin D, this increases for yearlings expected to mature at 500 kg to approximately 6000 IU/day of vitamin D.

The main deficiency signs relate to abnormal bone growth and skeletal development of youngstock. It is vital that pregnant and lactating mares and growing youngstock receive adequate levels of vitamin D to support bond growth and development. Deficiency signs include enlarged growth plates, loss of weight and bone demineralisation. Rickets in youngstock and osteomalacia in adult horses are both rare.

Vitamin D toxicity is the most common. Excess vitamin D accumulates over a period of weeks before causing toxicity symptoms, including abnormal deposition of calcium into soft tissues such as in the kidneys, heart valves and lungs. This calcium has been resorbed from bone within the horse's skeleton and so bones also become soft and brittle making them more likely to break or fracture.

The suggested safe level is 44 IU/kg bodyweight per day. (NRC, 1987).

# Vitamin E

Vitamin E is possibly the most important antioxidant vitamin, playing an essential role in the 'mopping up' of free radicals and therefore protecting cells from damage. As previously mentioned, free radicals are naturally produced during metabolic processes and have to be removed before they harm cells. Vitamin E is found within cells lipid membranes where it carries out its protective function. It is thought to boost the immune system and is an important anticoagulant reducing abnormal blood clotting within the body helping to keep blood vessels free from blockages. It also has a role in the release of energy from feed.

Vitamin E consists of a group of related substances that exist in a number of different forms, known as tocopherols and tocotrienols. The most important of these are the tocopherols of which alpha-tocopherol is the most significant within the horse's body. Green leafy plants are good sources of vitamin E.

Vitamin E is relatively unstable and in high moisture feeds such as haylage and silage vitamin E activity is very low. Biological activity of vitamin E is most usually expressed as IU or international units and 1 mg of dl-alpha- tocopherol acetate is equivalent to 1 IU vitamin E. However, another study found that the oral and natural form d-alpha-tocopherol was the most effective form of vitamin E.

Vitamin E interacts with glutathione peroxidase which contains the trace mineral selenium and these two compounds act synergistically. Vitamin C also has potent antioxidant activities, and in fact vitamin C is used in the regeneration process of vitamin E. Horses fed higher levels of oil or fat will benefit from additional vitamin E owing to the increased requirement for antioxidants. It is also recommended for improvement of reproductive function. Vitamin E is not stored in sufficient amounts within the horse's body for horses. Horses in hard work have increased requirements for vitamin E and vitamin E content in a feed is often a good indicator of its nutritional quality for performance and breeding horses. Vitamin E levels fall quickly as moisture levels in compound or cereal feeds increase and processing of cereals and poor storage of compound feeds will reduce vitamin E activity. Horses fed higher levels of oil will require additional vitamin E in the ration.

The daily requirement for a 500 kg horse at maintenance is 500 IU vitamin E/day, in medium work, 800 IU/day and hard work 1000 IU/day as suggested by NRC 2007.

1 IU of vitamin E is equivalent to 1 mg of alpha-tocopherol acetate (as above).

A deficiency of vitamin E may result in several equine diseases including equine motor neurone disease (EMND) and equine degenerative myeloencephalopathy (EDM). As yet there has been no scientific proof that vitamin E (and selenium) helps rhabdomyolysis or tying up, although this combination is often fed to horses with a history of this condition.

There are few reports of vitamin E toxicity or hypervitaminosis E in horses. It seems that vitamin E has a higher safer level of intake than the other fat soluble vitamins. The suggested safe level is 1000 IU/kgDM (NRC, 1987).

## Vitamin K

Vitamin K is actually a group of compounds but the two most common forms are vitamin K1, phylloquinone, and vitamin K2, menaquinone.

Normally, vitamin K2 is produced by the microorganisms in the horse's hindgut and this should be enough to meet the horse's requirements. Vitamin K is required for blood clotting, but as yet no requirement has been established in horses. Vitamin K is often used to help reduce or prevent exercise induced pulmonary haemorrhage (EIPH), although further research is required.

Research has also shown that vitamin K is important for bone development and growth. Some horses may have enough vitamin K in the ration for blood clotting, but lack enough for efficient bone metabolism. Although there are no estimated NRC requirements for vitamin K, is generally thought to be 10 mg/day.

## WATER SOLUBLE VITAMINS

Water soluble vitamins include vitamin B complex and vitamin C. Because they dissolve easily in water (hence the term water soluble) they are not stored in any great quantities in the horse's tissues and are easily lost from the horse's body via urine. An exception to this rule is vitamin B12, which is mainly stored in the liver. Horses therefore need a regular supply of most of these vitamins even though B vitamins are required in minute amounts. All water soluble vitamins are organic compounds but are actually chemically unrelated. B vitamins are often broadly described as metabolic cofactors that are mostly involved in the energy production process within cells. Vitamin B12 and folic acid are also involved in cell division. Many B complex vitamins work together, i.e. synergistically; however a deficiency of one will result in specific symptoms. Due to their different chemistry, water soluble vitamins are absorbed directly into the portal blood supply following digestion.

Water soluble vitamins with the exception of vitamins C and B12 are usually supplied in adequate amounts in good quality forage. However, most B vitamins are made within the horse's caecum and colon by microorganisms. These, in addition to dietary intake from forage and feed in normal circumstances, should be enough to meet requirements. However, for horses under stress or receiving antibiotics, production of these B vitamins may be compromised at a time when requirements are increased and there will be a need to supplement these horses.

## Vitamin C

Vitamin C or ascorbic acid is essential for collagen synthesis, a major structural protein in the horse's body. Vitamin C has a long list of different functions within the body. It is also important for growth and repair of body tissues, including bones and reproduction. Vitamin C helps to promote wound healing and is involved in red blood cell production and aids iron absorption. Vitamin C is another important antioxidant and is vital for helping regenerate vitamin E. It is thought to have powerful immune boosting properties as it helps white blood cells fight diseases. This important vitamin helps the horse's body to absorb folic acid and iron and aids in the energy production process. In humans vitamin C is also thought to lessen the duration of viral infections and is important for sperm health.

Under normal circumstances, horses do not need supplemental vitamin C as it is synthesised from glucose via a series of reactions in the horse's liver; humans appear to have lost the ability to do this. However, horses that are under increased stress such as occurs in those in hard work or growing rapidly, vitamin C supplementation may be beneficial. This seems to be particularly helpful in reducing shipping fever in horses when fed for five days at a rate of 5 g for youngstock and 10 g for adult horses, prior to transport. Feeding vitamin C continuously may not be advisable as horses may lose their ability to make their own and further research is required.

For horses in prolonged high intensity training vitamin C supplementation for short durations may be beneficial in helping to stabilise cell membranes and nutritionally support the immune system. The respiratory system seems to particularly benefit from vitamin C supplementation and horses with a compromised respiratory system may benefit from 10 mg vitamin C per day.

# B complex vitamins

- B1 – (thiamine)
- B2 – (riboflavin)
- B6 – (pyridoxine)
- Pantothenic acid
- Niacin (nicotinic acid)
- Folate
- B12 (cyanocobalamin)
- Biotin.

B complex vitamins are generally required for metabolism of carbohydrates, proteins and fats and are normally synthesised by the healthy microbes within the hindgut. Healthy horses on good quality forage are unlikely to be deficient, but horses in hard work, post viral or in stressful situations may respond to B vitamin supplementation. The injection of B vitamins, including vitamin B12 has not been shown to improve performance. Vitamin B12 is produced in the hindgut if there is enough cobalt in the diet.

## *Biotin*

Biotin is a B vitamin that has received much attention over the years for its effect on hoof growth and quality. Studies have shown its benefits in other species, although there are several other nutrients important for good hoof growth of which biotin is only one. For horses, long term use of biotin supplements over six to nine months or longer may help horses with poor quality hoof horn. Supplementation with 20 mg biotin daily did improve the quality of hoof horn but not the growth rate of the hoof wall.

Biotin is generally required as a coenzyme for several carboxylase enzymes that are involved in making fatty acids, glucose synthesis (gluconeogenesis) and amino acid metabolism. Biotin is also essential for cell proliferation. (See diet related problems, chapter 12 for more information.)

## *Folate (folic acid)*

Folate is important for cell growth, DNA and methionine synthesis. Folate is actually a general term given to the synthetic form, i.e. folic acid and the naturally occurring folate form, which have slightly different structures. Horses grazing fresh forage have higher amounts of serum folate than those eating conserved forage and/or cereal based hard feeds. Horses in training without access to fresh pasture may well have lower serum folate levels.

Lactating mares and foals may benefit from folate supplementation particularly if access to fresh pasture is limited. The folic acid level in milk falls through the first three months of lactation. As foals begin to eat green forage folic acid levels build up again in the body.

### Requirements of the other B vitamins

B vitamins are found in good quality forage and the germ of cereals. Horses in hard work, receiving antibiotic therapy or those on high concentrate rations may have impaired hindgut fermentation and may benefit from B vitamin supplementation.

NRC 2007 requirements for thiamine have been estimated for a 500 kg horse at maintenance as 30 mg/day. This rises to 62.5 mg/day for horses in hard work.

NRC 2007 requirements for riboflavin have been estimated for a 500 kg horse at maintenance as 20 mg/day. This rises to 25 mg/day for horses in hard work.

Information concerning requirements for vitamins B6, B12 and pantothenic acid is extremely limited.

Vitamin B12 is not present in plants but is made by hindgut microorganisms in the horse. Cobalt is required for vitamin B12 synthesis as mentioned earlier and supplementing 15 mg/day of cobalt in the diet has been shown to increase serum vitamin B12. No deficiency or toxicity of vitamin B12 in horses has been shown.

B vitamins may be supplemented for horses in hard work, that are stressed or post viral.

## Are vitamin supplements required?

Horses have requirements for all vitamins, but many of these are made within the horse's body. The amount required would depend upon several factors including:

- Reproductive status
- Age
- Bodyweight
- Temperament
- Workload
- Level of stress.
- Health status.

Before buying vitamin supplements for horses, it is important to take into account the amount of vitamins already contained in the horse's diet. Most compound feeds for performance horses and breeding stock will contain high levels of vitamins and if the feed is fed at the recommended rate or slightly above, then horses will not generally need further supplementation. However, if other factors, such as stress, illness, poor and/or inadequate forage or feed or reduced graying is present, a supplement may be helpful.

Horses on low amounts of feed or low level rations such as for breaking, or overweight horses in work will need vitamin and mineral supplementation. In general, feeding excessive amounts of vitamins in the hope of improving performance is not recommended.

---

**Summary points**

- Vitamins are required in minute quantities for optimum health of the horse, hence they are known as micronutrients.
- Vitamins are organic compounds that are either supplied in the horse's diet or the horse can make within the body, mostly within the hindgut.
- Vitamins are organic substances and are often unstable and therefore easily destroyed.
- Vitamins are grouped into two broad categories namely fat soluble (A,D,E and K) and water soluble (C and B group).
- Vitamin D is known as the sunshine vitamin. It is surprisingly present in higher concentrations in cut dried forages than in fresh pasture.
- Horses are able to make vitamin D from another provitamin, which is formed within the horse's skin in the presence of UV light.
- Horses that are out in sunlight for several hours daily or that are fed sun-dried hay in significant quantities are unlikely to be deficient in vitamin D.
- Permanently stabled horses on low forage rations will need vitamin D.
- Vitamin E is possibly the most important antioxidant vitamin.
- Vitamin E is relatively unstable and in high moisture feeds such as haylage, vitamin E activity is very low.
- Vitamin K is required for blood clotting, but as yet no requirement has been established in horses.
- Water soluble vitamins (except vitamin C and B12) are usually supplied in adequate amounts in good quality forage.
- Most B vitamins are made within the horse's caecum and colon by micro-organisms living there.
- B complex vitamins are generally required for the metabolism of carbohydrates, proteins and fats.
- For horses, long term use of biotin supplements over six to nine months or longer may help horses with poor quality hoof horn.
- B vitamins are found in good quality forage and the germ of cereals.
- Horses in hard work, receiving antibiotic therapy or post viral or those on high concentrate rations may benefit from B vitamin supplementation.

# Minerals

Minerals are inorganic substances that are naturally found in rocks, soil and water. Minerals are elements, i.e. they consist of only one type of atom. Plants such as grass take up these minerals via the root transport system from the soil and horses grazing them thereby take minerals into the body. Minerals remain as ash when all the carbon, hydrogen and nitrogen have been removed from food via burning in oxygen in a bomb calorimeter.

The horse's body contains roughly 22 known minerals most of which are thought to be essential for life. There may be as many as five more that are essential for metabolism but data is currently very limited. It is thought that minerals make up approximately 4% of the bodyweight of the horse. Table 5.1 shows the minerals and their sources and functions.

Minerals can be grouped according to the relative amounts required in the diet, namely macrominerals or microminerals (trace minerals). Macrominerals are generally needed in grams (g) or milligrams (mg) in the diet and microminerals in much smaller amounts such as micrograms (µg) or parts per million (ppm). Macrominerals and microminerals (ppm) are shown in Table 5.2.

Potassium, sodium and chloride are also known as the major electrolytes or body salts (see Chapter 8).

Some minerals are present in the body and are present as environmental contaminants including arsenic, vanadium, tin, silicon, nickel, boron, lead and cadmium. Once consumed, minerals can be difficult to remove from the body. Minerals that can dissolve in water may be excreted in the urine and others are evacuated in the droppings, however toxicity symptoms may result from over- supplementation or from injecting, e.g. iron.

Minerals are present either as components of biological molecules such as haemoglobin (iron), enzymes, the skeleton (calcium/

**Table 5.1** Minerals sources and functions.

| MAJOR MINERALS | | | |
|---|---|---|---|
| Ca Calcium | 98% of body Ca is found in skeleton and teeth<br>Blood clotting<br>Nerve and muscle function<br>Lactation | Alfalfa<br>Limestone flour<br>Green forage<br>Sugar beet | Bone problems<br>Rickets (young)<br>Osteomalacia (old)<br>Nutritional secondary hyperparathyroidism (Big head disease)<br>Enlarged joints<br>Tying up |
| P Phosphorus | 85% of body P is found in skeleton and teeth<br>Energy production<br>Enzyme systems | Cereals | Bone problems<br>Rickets (young)<br>Osteomalacia (old)<br>Reduced or depraved appetite.<br>Decreased growth |
| Mg Magnesium | 60–70% of body Mg found in skeleton and teeth<br>Enzyme systems | Alfalfa<br>Linseed | Weakness in limbs<br>Muscular tremors<br>Ataxia<br>Sweating |
| Na (Sodium)<br>Cl (Chloride)<br>K (Potassium) | Body fluid regulation<br>Muscle and nerve function<br>Acid base balance | Grass<br>Hay<br>Salt lick (NaCl only)<br>Horses have a specific appetite for salt | Sweating<br>Dehydration<br>Muscular weakness<br>Fatigue<br>Exhaustion<br>Depraved appetite |
| S Sulphur | Amino acid synthesis<br>Hoof and horn growth<br>Enzyme systems<br>Present in insulin | Grass | Poor hair and skin growth including hooves |
| MICROMINERALS | | | |
| Fe Iron | Haemoglobin syntheses<br>60% of body Fe is in haemoglobin<br>Enzyme activation | Most natural feeds | Anaemia<br>Weakness<br>Pale mucous membranes<br>Fatigue<br>Reduced growth<br>Mare's milk is low in Fe |
| Cu Copper | Haemoglobin synthesis<br>Pigmentation of hair<br>Cartilage and elastin production<br>Bone development<br>Interacts with S and Mo | Depends upon soil Cu content from which feed is grown.<br>High Mo reduces Cu availability. | Developmental orthopaedic disease<br>Intermittent diarrhoea<br>Loss of pigment in hair<br>Poor performance<br>Reduced growth |
| Zn Zinc | Cell metabolism<br>Enzyme activator<br>High Zn interferes with Cu utilisation<br>Immune system | Yeast<br>Cereals | Hair loss<br>Skin lesions<br>Reduced appetite<br>Reduced growth |

**Table 5.1** *Continued*

| MICROMINERALS | | | |
|---|---|---|---|
| I Iodine | Required for thyroxin hormone Controls metabolic rate | Most feeds Seaweed products | Infertility Goitre |
| Mo Molybdenum | Enzyme activator | Often excessive in soils and therefore pasture Forage High Mo affects Cu availability | Deficiency symptoms not seen |
| Se Selenium | Antioxidant Interacts with vitamin E | Pasture Soil content varies depending upon area Deficient areas are common USA has many areas where Se toxicity is common | Muscle disease Impaired cardiac function Respiratory problems Tying up |
| Mn Manganese | Carbohydrate, protein and fat metabolism Bone formation Lactation | Bran Grass (depending upon soil content) | Bone abnormalities Poor feed utilisation |
| Co Cobalt | Required for synthesis of vitamin B12 | Trace levels present in most feeds | Anaemia Weight loss Reduced growth |

**Table 5.2** Macrominerals and Microminerals.

| *Macrominerals – major minerals* | *Microminerals – trace minerals* |
|---|---|
| Calcium (Ca) | Copper (Cu) |
| Phosphorus (P) | Iron (Fe) |
| Sodium (Na) | Manganese (Mn) |
| Chlorine (Cl) (as chloride ions) | Zinc (Zn) |
| Potassium (K) | Iodine (I) (as iodide ions) |
| Magnesium (Mg) | Selenium (Se) |
| Sulphur | Molybdenum (Mo) |
| | Cobalt (Co) |
| | Chromium (Cr) |
| | *Fluorine* |
| | *Silicon* |

phosphorus) or hormones (iodine) or as ions in fluids helping to maintain homeostasis.

Some minerals are bound within larger molecules making them unavailable in feed. An example is phytate (inositol hexaphosphate) found in cereals and this binds calcium, zinc and iron making them less bioavailable to the horse.

## MACROMINERALS

### Calcium

The word calcium is derived from 'calx' the Greek word for lime or chalk. Calcium is the major mineral within the horse's body and the majority of it, around 99%, is found within the skeleton and teeth. The remaining 1% is found within the extracellular fluid in its ionic form.

Calcium provides strength to the skeleton as, in conjunction with phosphorus, both these macrominerals are found in the compound hydroxyapatite, $Ca_{10}(PO_4)_6(OH)_2$, the bone hardening compound. Bone also acts as a reserve for ionic calcium in fluids.

Calcium has the following functions:

- Major component of bone and teeth
- Transmission of nerve impulses
- Regulation of fluid balance, controlling water movement in and out of cells
- Enables normal clotting of blood
- Muscle contraction.

The skeleton acts as a reservoir of calcium as bone turnover is continual. Bone cells known as osteoblasts lay down new bone while other cells known as osteoclasts resorb it. During growth of foals and yearlings there is a net calcium gain but as horses finish growing the amount of calcium within the skeleton is relatively constant depending upon dietary intake.

Calcium is also vital for contraction and relaxation of muscles. An increase of calcium within cells is a trigger for muscle fibres to contract. The horse's heart is also a muscle and therefore calcium is required for the generation and control of the heartbeat. Calcium in body fluids is highly regulated within relatively narrow limits. This homeostasis is important and is regulated by parathyroid hormone (increases bone resorption), calcitonin (inhibits bone resorption) and vitamin D. These act upon the digestive tract, kidneys and the skeleton to alter the movement of calcium. Blood clotting is also affected if calcium levels fall.

Calcium in the diet is mostly absorbed in the small intestine (duodenum and jejunum). This absorption occurs both by passive diffusion and active transport (requiring energy). In general calcium salts are not readily soluble and certain factors can aid calcium absorption. Calcium binding protein is a vitamin D dependent protein in the cells of the intestinal wall, which carries calcium into the blood. If calcium levels fall, calcium binding protein synthesis is increased to aid calcium absorption from the digestive tract. Other factors, which enhance dietary calcium absorption, are lactose in mare's milk, which helps keep calcium in its soluble form, lysine and some other amino acids. The acidic environment of the stomach also helps to keep calcium in its soluble form.

Other factors may inhibit calcium absorption, such as phytate in cereal grains. Oxalates in wheat bran form an insoluble calcium oxalate salt, which is not absorbed. In addition, increased dietary calcium reduces the amount of calcium absorption. High phosphorus levels may also lead to changes in calcium metabolism but do not appear to affect calcium absorption per se. Calcium gluconate is a highly available source of calcium.

Calcium excretion occurs via the droppings, sweat and urine. Large amounts of calcium may be lost in horses' sweat at intensive work rates and high environmental temperatures. Calcium lost in horses' droppings represents that which has not been absorbed and also calcium from digestive enzymes, bile and dead or sloughed off cells from the wall of the digestive tract.

The main effect of calcium deficiency is seen in the skeleton. Bone becomes softer as the matrix becomes depleted of calcium. In young horses this may happen very quickly. Horses on calcium deficient diets often become lame with lameness shifting between different limbs. In young horses this loss of calcium and therefore bone strength is known as rickets and in older adult horses as osteomalacia.

Where calcium intake is normal but phosphorus intake is high, bone is again resorbed but much deeper within the bone resulting in replacement of bone tissue with fibrous connective tissue. This condition is known as nutritional secondary hyperparathyroidism. This effect occurs over the whole skeleton but is most visible in horses' heads where the head appears enlarged. This is consequently known as 'Big head' 'Bran' or 'Miller's' disease. The enlargement occurs in the upper and lower jaws and facial crest of horses. All cereal grains must be fortified or supplemented with calcium, as they are low in calcium and high in phosphorus. Compound feeds have calcium added but feeding unsupplemented straight cereals may result in calcium deficiency.

Calcium homeostasis maintains blood calcium levels within very narrow boundaries even when unbalanced rations are fed and so measuring total serum calcium in blood tests does not necessarily give an accurate view of total calcium status of the horse. The normal reference range for total serum calcium is 10.8–13.5 mg/dl serum. Blood results should be assessed alongside nutritional evaluation of the overall diet.

Calcium has been fed at levels as high as five times requirements without any harmful effects as long as the phosphorus intake is meeting requirements.

NRC 2007 states that a 500 kg horse at maintenance will require 20 g/day; in hard work this rises to 40 g/day. Foals to two year olds will need around 37–40 g/day to support skeletal growth. Lactating mares will need 60 g/day calcium at month one of lactation falling to 37 g/day at month six. Pregnant mares require 20 g/day for the first six months and then up to 36 g for the last three months of gestation.

## Phosphorus

Phosphorus is often considered together with calcium as both are involved in bone metabolism and control of blood phosphorus is similar to that for calcium. Roughly 85% of the body's phosphorus is found within bone, phosphorus is therefore essential for bone and teeth but it is also required to transmit the genetic code from one cell to another.

Phosphorus has the following functions:

- Major component of bone and teeth
- Helps to maintain blood pH – phosphates essential for buffering
- Component of phospholipids – transport of fats and fatty acids between tissues
- Component of RNA and DNA – essential for protein synthesis, transmission of genetic information
- Required for ADP and ATP the energy currency of all cells
- Component of myelin – a fatty sheath that surrounds nerve cells.

Phosphorus levels are regulated within the horse's body by excretion through the kidneys under the influence of parathyroid hormone, which increases phosphorus loss via the urine. Homeostasis for phosphorus appears less sensitive than for calcium.

Phosphorus absorption is more effective than calcium, but varies depending upon age of the horse, feed ingredients and the amount of phosphorus fed. Phosphorus absorption is reduced if dietary calcium levels are high and high levels of oxalates will also reduce phosphorus retention.

Phosphorus deficiency will result in ricket-like symptoms in younger horses and osteomalacia in older ones, although true phosphorus deficiency in horses is rare. Excessive dietary phosphorus reduces calcium absorption resulting in calcium deficiency and Nutritional Secondary Hyperparathyroidism (see Calcium deficiency above).

NRC 2007 states that a 500 kg horse at maintenance will require 14 g phosphorus/day; in hard work this rises to 29 g/day. Foals to two year olds will need around 20–22 g/day to support skeletal growth. Lactating mares will need 38 g/day phosphorus at month one of lactation falling to 23 g/day at month six. Pregnant mares require 14 g/day for the first six months and then up to 26 g for the last three months of gestation.

### Calcium:phosphorus ratio

Dietary calcium intake must always exceed phosphorus, otherwise calcium absorption is reduced and calcium deficiency may result. This means a minimum ratio of 1:1 Ca:P. Feeding large amounts of cereal grains or bran that have not been fortified/supplemented with calcium may result in a reverse Ca:P ratio as all cereal grains and bran contain substantially higher levels of phosphorus than calcium (see Appendix 2). Feeding unfortified cereals with low calcium forage will also result in calcium deficiency. Aiming for a calcium to phosphorus ratio of 1.5:1 Ca:P is ideal.

## Magnesium

The majority of magnesium is found within the skeleton. The content of most feeds that horses consume is 0.1–0.3%, horses require 0.1% magnesium in the diet and so the needs of most horses are met by common equine diets. Grass contains chlorophyll, which contains magnesium, and so reasonable forage intakes should meet magnesium requirements.

Neither magnesium deficiency nor excess has been reported extensively in horses fed natural feeds. Magnesium is absorbed mainly in the upper area of the small intestine by diffusion, both ordinary and facilitated. If magnesium intake is low, then absorption from the digestive tract is increased. Absorption of magnesium is increased by vitamin D and reduced by phytate (see calcium) and fatty acids.

Sixty per cent of body magnesium is found in bone, 20% in muscle, 1% in extracellular fluid and the remainder in other soft tissues. Magnesium occurs as part of cell membranes and is an essential activator of many enzymes. It is required for all enzyme systems that use the body's universal energy currency, i.e. ATP (adenosine triphosphate). In addition it is involved in some protein synthesis, muscle contraction and the transmission of nerve impulses.

Magnesium is the most abundant intracellular ion and most bone magnesium is locked into apatite in the skeleton. Low dietary magnesium therefore is more likely to result in muscle problems such as tiredness, work intolerance, muscle tremors and ataxia. Horses may also be over-excited, but this symptom on its own is unlikely to be a result of magnesium deficiency. Magnesium is absorbed mainly from the small intestine with smaller amounts being absorbed from the large intestine of horses.

Acute magnesium deficiency has occasionally occurred in heavily lactating mares and during acute stress and/or during long distance transport when horses have not been fed for many hours. Magnesium deficiency problems are much greater in cows as horses absorb this important mineral much more efficiently. Rare cases of magnesium deficiency are shown by neuromuscular excitability, i.e. muscle tremors, ataxia or wobbly gait and hot temperament or hyper-excitability. Horses may not tolerate work at all.

Magnesium deficiency is so rare it is not routinely tested for and it is difficult to establish in blood tests, as the plasma levels tend to remain relatively constant, therefore muscle biopsies are preferred as they are more accurate. If low muscle magnesium is found then it may be supplemented, but excessive magnesium intake is definitely not recommended. This results in changes to the pH in the intestine and may result in the formation of intestinal stones and/or metabolic disorders.

To date, scientific trials evaluating magnesium toxicity have not been carried out. The NRC has estimated a maximum tolerable magnesium intake at 0.8% of the diet. Magnesium supplementation of horses' rations to help calm horses and for barefoot horses is rapidly on the increase and this could certainly result in increased intakes over the period of supplementation. Magnesium supplements tend to be given over long periods of time and this should be avoided unless dietary magnesium evaluation shows low dietary magnesium intakes.

Normal serum magnesium levels range from 18 μg/dl to 35 μg/dl (NRC 2005).

NRC 2007 states that a 500 kg horse at maintenance will require 7.5 g magnesium/day; in hard work this rises to 15 g/day. Foals to yearlings will need around 3–6 g/day to support skeletal growth. Working two year olds will need as much as 13 g magnesium/day. Lactating mares will need 11 g/day magnesium for the first two months of lactation falling to 10 g/day at month five. Pregnant mares require approximately 7.5 g/day throughout gestation.

## Potassium

The majority of body potassium is found within the cells, particularly skeletal muscle cells, bound to proteins and phosphate; 75% of the body's potassium is found within skeletal muscle cells. Less than 1.5% of body potassium is found outside cells in the surrounding extracellular fluid. Similar to sodium, potassium is required for maintaining fluid, electrolyte and acid–base balance. It is also essential for the sending of impulses along nerve fibres and contraction of muscles. Potassium salts are mainly organic and are important for osmotic pressure and, as such, any that leaks from within cells is quickly pumped back in. Potassium will therefore determine the volume of individual cells. This is vital to help maintain the differential between the composition of fluids inside and outside of cells on which so many of the cells' functions depend. As potassium is found within cells, sodium is typically found outside in the fluid bathing them.

Potassium is readily absorbed from the upper small intestine and hindgut.

Forage is a rich source of potassium generally containing 1–2%. Thus high levels of forage will greatly exceed the requirements. Cereal grains contain roughly 0.3–0.4% potassium.

Excretion of potassium from the kidneys increases when horses exercise. If the horse is also sweating then potassium losses can be high. Body potassium levels must be carefully regulated to maintain low levels within the plasma and other extracellular fluid (i.e. fluid found outside cells) and much higher levels inside cells. If potassium intake is high, and the extracellular fluid potassium levels start to rise, then horses will excrete more potassium through the kidneys into the urine and small amounts in the faeces. Conversely if potassium intake is low the horse is not as good at conserving it.

NRC 2007 states that a 500 kg horse at maintenance will require 25 g potassium/day; in hard work this rises to 40–50 g/day. Foals to weanlings will require about 10–17 g potassium/day and two year olds will need around 25 g/day to support skeletal growth and work for racing thoroughbreds. Lactating mares will need 45–48 g/day potassium at monthsone to three of lactation falling to 34 g/day at month six. Pregnant mares require 25 g/day throughout gestation.

## Sodium and chloride

These two minerals are usually found together as sodium chloride or salt. Chloride normally accompanies sodium as the anion chloride. Salt has long been thought of as a valuable commodity, in fact roman soldiers were paid a 'salarium' with which to buy salt. Many wild herbivores in arid geographical areas have sources of salt, which they return to when the need arises. Sodium is often required in order to remove or excrete excessive levels of potassium from the natural herbage diet. It is interesting that sodium does not seem to be essential for plants.

Dietary sodium intake for horses is relatively low as natural feedstuffs are low in salt (often less than 0.1%). Salt is often added to compound feeds at rates of 0.5–1% and free choice salt licks are often made available for horses. Both sodium and chloride are easily absorbed from the digestive tract. Sodium absorption is mostly active and requires energy. Chloride is mainly absorbed passively along electrochemical gradients in the small intestine. Sodium and chloride are also secreted into the small intestine via digestive juices and saliva and much of this is reabsorbed in the hindgut.

Each gram of sodium chloride or common salt contains 17.1 mmol sodium and is the main cation in extracellular fluids (ECF), i.e. those that surround and bathe cells, and comprises around 90% of the cations in blood. The average sodium concentration in ECF is 140 mmol/l. A 500 kg horse would have an ECF volume of approximately 100 l.

Approximately half the body's sodium is dissolved in the ECF. And about 40% is found in bone. Of this 40%, about half is mobilisable and the remaining is thought to be inaccessible deep within the mineral lattice. The remainder is found within the digesta in the gut, blood, muscle and skin.

Sodium is required for:

- Normal functioning of the central nervous system
- Maintenance of extracellular fluid and therefore blood volume
- Osmotic regulation of body fluids
- Maintenance of electrochemical gradients across cell membranes
- Maintenance of acid–base balance.

Electrochemical gradients are vital for the transmission of nerve impulses and contraction of muscle fibres. They are also important for the movement of substances such as glucose into and out of cells across the cell membrane and against concentration gradients such as are required in the digestive tract and kidneys. In fact the movement of ions across electrochemical gradients and the continuous maintenance of vital gradients requires a great deal of energy from ATP.

Sodium levels must be maintained in the blood at a constant level and body sodium balance is therefore closely regulated. Sodium is not stored and is normally lost through sweat, faeces and urine. Kidneys excrete excess dietary sodium above that lost in sweat and faeces. Basically, the rate at which sodium is excreted from the kidneys is dependent upon the speed of filtration in the glomerulus and the amount of resorption in the kidney tubules. This provides great flexibility in adjustment of plasma sodium levels. The mechanism for this is complicated and the hormone aldosterone, secreted from the cortex of the adrenal glands, plays a major role. Excretion of chloride also occurs mainly through the kidneys.

Dietary salt is mostly required for exercising/sweating horses to meet losses. However, digesta within the large intestine act as a reservoir for water, sodium, potassium and chloride and this helps to reduce the chance of low plasma sodium levels (hyponatraemia) occurring.

NRC 2007 states that a 500 kg horse at maintenance will require 10 g sodium/day; in hard work this rises to 25–40 g/day. Foals to yearlings will need around 4–7 g/day and hard working two year olds will as much as need 22–35 g sodium/day. Lactating mares will need about 13 g/day sodium for the first two months of lactation falling to 11.5 g/day at month six. Pregnant mares require approximately 10–11 g/day throughout gestation.

# MICROMINERALS

## Iron

Iron is a trace mineral that has been recognised as a required nutrient for horses for over 100 years. It is an essential part of the important haemoglobin molecule in blood, which contains about 0.34% iron. Blood therefore accounts for roughly 60% of the body's iron content. Some iron is also found in myoglobin within the horse's muscles (about 20%) and myoglobin has a greater affinity for oxygen than haemoglobin. The remaining iron is used in enzymes (mainly cytochromes) or is stored within the horse's liver.

Iron is used for:

- Red blood cell synthesis (70–90%)
- Myoglobin synthesis in muscle cells
- Production of cytochromes in mitochondria
- Immune function
- Hormone and neurotransmitter synthesis.

Haemoglobin in red blood cells carries oxygen from the lungs to the body tissues enabling cellular respiration to take place. This is vital for horses, as oxygen carrying capacity is required to supply muscles with oxygen to burn fuel for work.

Iron is absorbed from the small intestine in the ferrous state and once inside the body the horse holds on to this tenaciously. Iron absorption from the small intestine will increase when horses need more and the percentage absorbed will decrease when horses need less. This is a highly effective regulating mechanism. Iron absorption is, however, reduced by interactions with other minerals such as excessive dietary intakes of copper, manganese, cadmium and zinc.

Iron is conserved to a huge extent by horses and iron within haemoglobin (from red blood cells which are renewed roughly every 120 days), is recycled. This means that body iron is retained as much as possible and the recycling and regulating processes are highly efficient.

Forage usually contains between 100 and 200 mg/kg of iron although this may be as high as 400 mg/kg. Iron levels may be particularly high in acidic topsoil and these should be limed to adjust the pH. Cereals contain 30–90 mg/kg of inorganic iron some of which may also be bound to phytate making it unavailable for absorption. This shows that equine feedstuffs under normal circumstances should meet the dietary needs even for racehorses in training. Foals could be more susceptible to low iron as mare's milk is low in iron, decreasing as lactation progresses; even so clinical iron deficiency in foals is rare. This is because foals are born with high levels of iron in the plasma.

Iron deficiency tends to occur in horses owing to blood loss. This could be acute following a severe injury or chronic owing to intestinal parasites, lice infestation, bleeding in the lungs or gastric ulcers. Initially iron will be depleted from the horse's liver, spleen and bone marrow and this all occurs before anaemia symptoms are observed. Anaemia causes a decrease in the horse's capacity for work and generally increases fatigue. Iron supplements should not be given to horses unless confirmed iron deficiency anaemia has been diagnosed. Haematinics (iron tonics) or intramuscular iron injections are often given to horses to 'improve' performance. If there is no iron deficiency these will at best have no effect and at worst be harmful possibly causing iron toxicosis. Iron toxicosis is much more common than iron deficiency.

The horse's body is unable to excrete excess iron, if this is given orally as a supplement or paste then horses will reduce the amount of iron absorbed from the small intestine. However, if injected, the self-regulating mechanism is bypassed, giving no protection from possible iron toxicosis. In addition, excess iron in the body increases the horse's susceptibility to bacterial infections. Bacteria need iron to multiply and when they invade, horses are able to reduce available iron as one of their defence mechanisms against infection.

Blood tests are routinely used to determine iron status in horses, namely haematocrit (packed cell volume) and haemoglobin levels, both of which are fairly insensitive, that is neither falls until iron deficiency is fully established. Also horses store a large number of red blood cells in the spleen. During exercise, the spleen contracts and releases many of these stored red blood cells into the blood and this may increase the haematocrit and haemoglobin levels by as much as 50%. The plasma concentration of ferritin is the best indicator of iron status in horses.

Iron and copper compete for the same site of absorption in the small intestine and so high dietary iron levels can reduce copper absorption. Copper deficiency may result in nutritional anaemia. Feeding more iron will further reduce copper absorption and therefore exacerbate copper deficiency induced nutritional anaemia.

NRC 2007 states that a 500 kg horse at maintenance will require 400 mg iron/day; in hard work this rises to 500 mg/day. Foals to yearlings will need around 200–400 mg/day. Working two year olds will need as much as 537 mg iron/day. Lactating mares will need 625 mg/day iron through lactation. Pregnant mares require approximately 400–500 mg/day throughout gestation.

## Copper

Copper deficiency is well known in animals, resulting in anaemia and failure to grow and mature. Copper is essential for haemoglobin synthesis and many copper dependent enzymes are involved in production of elastic connective tissue. Copper is also required for mobilisation of body iron stores and melanin (hair pigmentation) production. Copper is vital for production of cartilage in youngstock.

Copper content of pasture varies depending upon the soil where it is grown. Copper is found mainly tightly bound to proteins known as metalloproteins, which are involved in many reactions both inside and outside the cell. Of the total body copper approximately 40% is found in skeletal muscle, the remainder is in liver (where it is stored), brain and blood (in red cells and as caeruloplasmin in plasma). Caeruloplasmin is required for iron metabolism converting ferrous iron to its ferric state, which then binds to transferrin and enters the cells. Ferrous iron ($Fe_2^+$) is soluble whereas ferric iron ($Fe_3^+$) is insoluble. Copper is vital for optimal growth of the foetus and foal (see Chapter 12). Copper is absorbed in the small intestine but interactions with dietary zinc and iron may reduce uptake.

Copper interacts with many other minerals including molybdenum, sulphur, iron, selenium and zinc. It is thought that horses can tolerate higher levels of molybdenum in the diet than ruminants, without affecting affect copper availability, however there is some debate about this.

Horses can tolerate relatively high dietary copper intakes and the maximum tolerable intake for horses is estimated at 250 mg/kg of ration.

High copper levels such as often found in same mineral blocks for breeding stock are very dangerous for sheep and to lesser extent for cattle. Care should be taken when using them.

NRC 2007 states that a 500 kg horse at maintenance will require 100 mg copper/day; in hard work this rises to 125 mg/day. Foals to yearlings will need around 42–97 mg/day. Working two year olds will need as much as 107 mg copper/day. Lactating mares will need 125 mg/day copper through lactation. Pregnant mares require approximately 100 mg/day for the first eight months of gestation rising to 125 mg/day from month nine.

# Zinc

Zinc is a component of many enzymes involved in tissue growth, wound healing, immune function and protein synthesis and is therefore widely distributed around the body with higher amounts found in hair, bones and skin. Zinc is absorbed in the small intestine and this is increased when dietary zinc is lower. Zinc deficiency causes reduced appetite, reduced fertility, poor wound healing, reduced growth and DOD (developmental orthopaedic disease). Zinc storage in the body is low and therefore daily dietary intake is important. Horses appear to tolerate high levels of dietary zinc.

Zinc may be found in a number of molecules including zinc sulphate, zinc oxide and zinc carbonate all of which are absorbed at different rates. The absorption of zinc may vary from 5% to 90%, whereas the absorption of calcium may vary from 10% to 40%. Supplementary zinc should be balanced with copper in a ration of 4:1.

NRC 2007 states that a 500 kg horse at maintenance will require 400 mg zinc/day; in hard work this rises to 500 mg/day. Foals to yearlings will need around 168–388 mg/day. Working two year olds will need as much as 430 mg zinc/day. Lactating mares will need 625 mg/day zinc through lactation. Pregnant mares require approximately 400 mg/day throughout gestation.

## Manganese

Manganese is essential for carbohydrate and fat metabolism and is a component of many enzymes; it is also important for production of joint cartilage being required for synthesis of chondroitinsulphate. Manganese is one of the least toxic of all the microminerals. Manganese deficiency is rare as it is widely available in equine feedstuffs.

NRC 2007 states that a 500 kg horse at maintenance will require 400 mg manganese/day; in hard work this rises to 500 mg/day. Foals to yearlings will need around 168–388 mg/day. Working two year olds will need as much as 430 mg manganese/day. Lactating mares will need 500 mg/day manganese through lactation. Pregnant mares require approximately 400 mg/day throughout gestation.

## Selenium

Selenium is a component of glutathione peroxidase, an important antioxidant; it plays a role in the control of thyroid hormones and is important for immune function. Selenium is thought to have potent anticancer properties in humans. Equine feedstuffs vary in selenium content from 0.01 to 0.3 mg/kg depending upon soil selenium content and acidity of the soil where the feed was grown. Some plants known as accumulator plants can store selenium in high concentrations and may cause toxicity when eaten by horses although this is not a problem in the United Kingdom. There are selenium deficient areas in the UK including parts of Scotland and determination of selenium status of pasture is important. Excess selenium is stored in the liver and can quickly become toxic if fed at ten times the recommended amount; this gives little margin for error. Over-supplementation is therefore possible when compound feeds are fed with additional selenium containing supplements. Large doses of selenium can be fatal to horses. Chronic selenium toxicity known as alkali disease results firstly in fatigue followed by cracking of the hoof and coronet band prior to hoof loss and is obviously life threatening. There have been several cases of deaths of horses caused by acute Se overdose including 21 polo ponies in Florida in 2009, who were accidentally administered with a toxic overdose of selenium. Mane and tail hair can also fall out. Selenium deficiency results in weakness and muscle disease, reduced performance and poor growth.

There is a narrow safety margin between Se requirements and toxic levels. Overdosing is therefore more likely. Selenium in forage and grains is normally present in its organic form as selenocystine, selenocysteine and selenomethionine. However, sodium selenite and sodium selenate are common inorganic sources in equine compound feeds.

Normal blood selenium values have been ascertained at 130–160 ng/ml.

NRC 2007 states that a 500 kg horse at maintenance will require 1.0 mg selenium/day; in hard work this rises to 1.25 mg/day. Foals to yearlings will need around 0.4–0.97 mg/day. Working two year olds will need 1.07 mg selenium/day. Lactating mares will need 1.25 mg/day selenium through lactation. Pregnant mares require approximately 1.0 mg/day throughout gestation.

## Iodine

Iodine is required for the synthesis of the thyroid hormones T3 triiodothyronine and T4 thyroxin and therefore most iodine is found within the thyroid gland. These thyroid hormones are heavily involved with regulating basal metabolism. A deficiency or excess of iodine results in similar symptoms, namely hypothyroidism, resulting in the characteristic enlargement of the thyroid gland or goitre. Seaweed and kelp may have iodine concentrations as high as 1850 mg/kgDM whereas most equine feedstuffs contain 0–2 mg/kg DM. Iodised or trace mineralised salt blocks contain roughly 70 mg/kg DM. The maximum tolerable intake of iodine is 5 mg/kg dietary intake. Breeding stock should not be fed seaweed or kelp as this can result in goitre in foals.

Iodine is found within the body in its ionic form iodide and is absorbed from the small intestine.

NRC 2007 states that a 500 kg horse at maintenance will require 3.5 mg iodine/day; in hard work this rises to 4.4 mg/day. Foals to yearlings will need around 1.5–3.4 mg/day. Working two year olds will as much as need 3.8 mg iodine/day. Lactating mares will need 4.4 mg/day iodine through lactation. Pregnant mares require approximately 3.5 mg/day for the first eight months of gestation rising to 4.0 mg from month nine.

## Chromium

Chromium plays an important role in carbohydrate and lipid metabolism. It works closely with insulin to facilitate the uptake of glucose into cells. In horses with insulin resistance (IR) chromium is of paramount importance. Without chromium, blood sugar levels stay elevated because the action of insulin is blocked and glucose is not transported into the cells.

Brewer's yeast is a good source of chromium, but chromium is not currently recognised as an additive to horse feed in Europe. It is therefore not generally available in equine compound feeds and supplements as no requirement has been determined. In addition, for horses with PSSM (polysaccharide storage myopoathy), which involves an abnormal sensitivity to insulin, additional chromium is not recommended.

## Silicon

Silicon is involved in formation of new bone and is an important constituent of connective tissue, cartilage and hyaluronic acid. Silicon is present mostly as silica and this is poorly absorbed. Sodium zeolite is a form that is more easily absorbed following breakdown in the stomach. Some research has indicated increased bone formation and reduced bone resorption when sodium zeolite is supplemented. This may be beneficial for young racehorses in training. As yet no dietary requirement for silicon has been determined but this could change in the near future.

## ORGANIC MICROMINERALS

The most common source of minerals in equine diets is found in the inorganic forms including carbonates, chlorides, oxides and sulphates, for example sodium chloride, calcium carbonate, iron sulphate. Availability of mineral ions from inorganic sources is variable. Oxides have the lowest availability and sulphates have the highest.

Organic mineral sources such as chelated minerals are therefore becoming more common as these are thought to be more available.

Chelated (sometimes referred to as bioplex) minerals have therefore received much attention and these are inorganic mineral ions that have been joined together with an amino acid, peptide, polysaccharide or propionate resulting in an organic structure.

Research has shown that chelated zinc, manganese and copper are 20–75% more available than the inorganic forms often added to horse feed and supplements. Selenium yeast is produced by a different method. Dried non-viable yeast is fermented with selenium enabling selenium to be incorporated into the organic material. Research has shown improved digestibility and retention with organic selenium yeast compared with the inorganic source, sodium selenite.

## Mineral interactions

Mineral levels vary tremendously in equine feedstuffs, particularly trace minerals. Research has shown that mineral concentrations of pasture appear to vary with the season, being higher in summer months and lower in autumn and consequently blood copper and zinc levels are highest in summer months. Blood iron levels seem highest during the spring. Except for copper, mineral levels appear significantly lower in winter than those in summer months.

In addition, pasture mineral levels may depend upon many other factors including:

• Region
• Grass variety and age
• Fertilisation history.

Minerals may compete with each other for absorption within the digestive tract. High calcium intakes may reduce the absorption of iron and magnesium and high zinc intakes may reduce the absorption of copper and iron. These are known as mineral interactions. Also high zinc levels may interfere with copper absorption and utilisation even though the copper requirements have been met in the diet. Iron and copper compete for the same site of absorption in the small intestine and so high dietary iron levels can reduce copper absorption, Selenium may be toxic in some regions such as in the USA and there is a relatively narrow safety margin between selenium requirements and toxic levels. Over-supplementation with selenium is therefore relatively common particularly when the pasture level is unknown and can cause severe health problems, even death. High levels of macrominerals such as calcium, will also affect how much phosphorus, magnesium, zinc and copper are absorbed from the diet.

An unbalanced ration can lead to deficiencies of some minerals, particularly microminerals even though requirements for all the minerals have theoretically been met in the diet.

The source of inorganic minerals in premixes used for compound feeds and supplements is also important. For example, sulphate sources tend to be more available than carbonates and oxides as they are more soluble, but sulphates can be damaging to vitamin A and thiamine in a premix. Chelated or organic trace minerals are therefore increasingly used instead.

Over-supplementation undertaken without nutritional or veterinary supervision may cause toxicities of some minerals and deficiencies of others and therefore advice should be taken.

---

**Summary points**

- Minerals are inorganic substances that are naturally found in rocks, soil and water.
- The horse's body contains roughly 22 known minerals most of which are thought to be essential for life.
- Minerals can be grouped according to the relative amounts required in the diet, namely macrominerals or microminerals (trace minerals).
- Potassium, sodium and chloride are also known as the major electrolytes.
- The horse's skeleton acts as an active reservoir of calcium as bone turnover is continual.
- Calcium homeostasis maintains blood calcium levels within very narrow boundaries.
- All cereal grains must be fortified or supplemented with calcium, as all cereals are low in calcium and high in phosphorus.
- Roughly 85% of the horse's body phosphorus is found within bone.
- Phosphorus is therefore essential for bone and teeth but it is also required to transmit the genetic code from one cell to another.
- Dietary calcium intake must always exceed phosphorus, otherwise calcium absorption is reduced and calcium deficiency will result.
- Magnesium is mostly found within the skeleton.
- The magnesium content of most feeds that horses consume is 0.1–0.3%, horses require 0.1% magnesium in the diet and so the needs of most horses are met by the diet.
- Forage is a rich source of potassium generally containing 1–2%.
- Dietary sodium intake for horses is relatively low as natural feedstuffs are low in salt (often less than 0.1%).
- Iron is conserved to a huge extent by the horse and the iron within haemoglobin (from red blood cells which are renewed roughly every 120 days), is recycled.
- Iodine deficiency and toxicity result in the same symptoms.
- Organic mineral sources such as chelated minerals are becoming more common in horse feeds as they are thought to be more available.

# Energy – Fuel for Life

Horses are mainly used for work or breeding. Horses traditionally worked in the fields as draft horses or were ridden as a main form of transport. Today, many horses are involved in major economic industries such as horse racing and breeding, show jumping, polo, dressage and three-day eventing, specifically for athletic performance. Other horses are mainly leisure animals used for performance, breeding and recreational purposes.

Energy is the most important aspect of the athletic horse's diet as the need for energy increases rapidly when horses work. Energy provides fuel for the working muscles and although not an actual nutrient, energy is chemically derived from nutrients such as carbohydrates (soluble and insoluble), i.e. including fibre, lipids/fats and, to a much lesser extent in the healthy horse, amino acids. Although energy cannot be seen it may be felt, for example as heat and also in physical movement or work. Horses need a certain amount of energy just for life, to walk around grazing and fuelling life processes (Figure 6.1). This is known as the energy requirement for maintenance $E_m$. Once horses begin exercising or working this energy requirement increases and is known as the energy requirement for work $E_w$. The harder the horse works the more energy is required and horses in very hard work such as racehorses in full training can be difficult to supply with all the energy they need and weight loss may result.

Horses undergoing very fast work for short speeds use energy differently from horses doing slower work over long periods such as endurance. Other horses also require large amounts of energy such as lactating mares in the first three months of lactation. They need nearly as much daily energy as racehorses in fast training. For example, a 500 kg horse in very fast work requires 34.5 Mcal per day whereas a 500 kg lactating mare requires 31.7 Mcal per day (NRC 2007 *Requirements of Horses* 6th revised edition).1 Mcal is a megacalorie and is equivalent

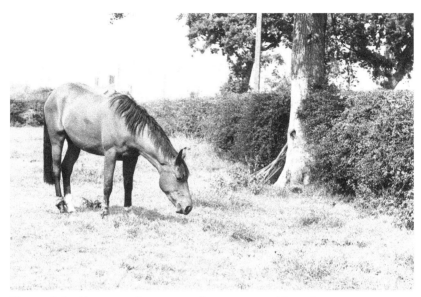

**Figure 6.1**   Horses need energy just for maintaining life and grazing.

to 1000 kilocalories (kcal). (To convert Mcal to MJ multiply by 4.184.)
The digestion of food results in energy substrates being absorbed into
the horse's body. The chemically bound energy from these substrates
must then be converted to mechanical energy for muscle contraction.

## ENERGY

Energy is defined as the ability to do work. It is mostly derived from
organic compounds from food, particularly carbohydrates, proteins
and fats/lipids. These compounds are derived from the chemical and
physical breakdown and absorption of ingested food within the gut.
These are then transported into the blood system and ultimately to
body cells including muscle cells. The horse obtains energy within
body cells from a chemical process known as cellular respiration, which
involves partial or complete oxidation of 'food' molecules absorbed
from the horse's digestive tract. Potential energy giving substrates for
work derived from the horse's diet include glucose, VFAs (volatile fatty
acids)' (acetic, propionic and butyric acids), fatty acids and amino acids
from proteins. Horses may also obtain energy from the metabolism of
stored carbohydrate (glycogen), fats (fat deposits) and body proteins
(particularly in very thin, starving horses). The breakdown of amino

acids for energy is accelerated when horses are in severe negative energy balance and horses use their own body tissues to supply the energy required to maintain life processes. The balance between carbohydrate and fat metabolism may be affected by the horse's diet, condition and physiological status.

The fate of different energy sources is shown in Figure 6.2.

Fat is the most concentrated source of energy providing the horse's body with almost twice as much energy as carbohydrates or protein.

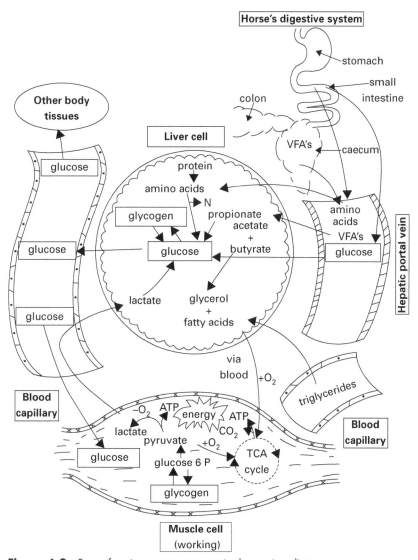

**Figure 6.2**  Fate of major energy sources in the equine diet.

All foods for horses contain a mixture of nutrients and the energy value will depend upon the amount of carbohydrates, fats and proteins within that food. Oils such as linseed or vegetable oil provide mainly fat while cereals provide a mix of carbohydrates, oils and protein.

## Glucose

The main substance oxidised within the horse's cells is glucose.

Glucose + Oxygen $\rightarrow$ Carbon dioxide + Water + Energy (673 kcal or 2800 kJ)

The amount of energy produced is approximately 673 kcal or 2800 kJ/mole of glucose. (A mole is a measure based upon the number of molecules it contains.)

In reality this chemical process is not simple and consists of a series of complex steps each speeded up by a specific enzyme taking place in all body cells. Many of these enzymes have cofactors such as thiamine, riboflavin, niacin and pantothenic acid, i.e. B vitamins that are essential for energy metabolism.

The chemical process is known as glycolysis or the glycolytic pathway, which converts glucose to a substance called pyruvate. Pyruvate then enters the TCA cycle (tricarboxylic acid) (also known as Krebs cycle or citric acid cycle) within the mitochondria of the cell. In the presence of oxygen, pyruvate enters the mitochondria where it is converted to a substance called acetyl-CoA (see Figure 6.3 energy production). Alternatively, pyruvate may be reduced to lactate in the cytoplasm of the cell. In the absence of oxygen lactate may accumulate in the cytoplasm producing increased acidity from lactic acid, causing muscle fatigue following strenuous exercise.

The TCA cycle is the final common energy pathway for not only carbohydrates, but also for lipids and the carbon skeleton of amino acids.

This is a complex series of reactions dependent upon the energy substrates and amount of oxygen available and the intensity of physical exercise being undertaken.

As mentioned above glucose may be derived from digestion and absorption from the gut or from its storage form in the body called glycogen. Circulating blood glucose may therefore have been derived from either the diet or gluconeogenesis or glycogenolysis in the liver. Red blood cells and brain cells depend almost entirely upon glucose as an energy source.

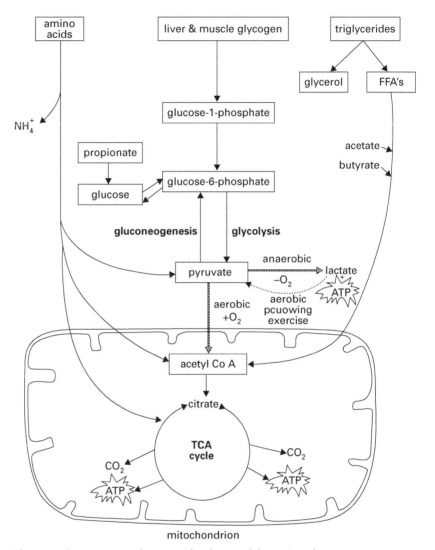

**Figure 6.3**  Energy production – glycolysis and the TCA cycle.

## Glycogen

Glycogen is stored in the horse's muscle and liver cells and consists of long chains of glucose linked together. When glucose is stored as glycogen it is stored with three times its own weight of water. In addition, the formation of glycogen from glucose requires two molecules of ATP for every molecule of glucose added to the chain.

Glycogen storage within the horse's body is limited and when horses ingest more carbohydrate than they need stores of muscle and liver glycogen are full. Further excess glucose is then converted to and stored as fat. This is achieved by the breakdown of excess glucose to pyruvate, which is then made available for fat synthesis for storage. The amount of glycogen stored in the thoroughbred is approximately 4.5 kg or 75 MJ. Fat is stored as triglycerides in much larger quantities than carbohydrate mainly in adipose tissue under the skin with some surrounding the internal organs and a small amount marbling the muscle. The thoroughbred has approximately 25 kg of fat stored, which is approximately 640 MJ. When this stored fat is needed by the horse, the triglycerides are broken down to long chain fatty acids and glycerol and released into the horse's bloodstream for use.

Short chain fatty acids from VFAs are produced from fibre fermentation in the horse's hindgut. It is estimated that horses on a primarily hay diet may derive as much as 80% of their required energy from VFAs.

Glycogen may be rapidly turned back into glucose by hydrolysis, for use by the horse allowing blood glucose levels to be maintained within a narrow range by conversion of excess circulating glucose to glycogen (glycogenesis) and by reconversion of stored glycogen to glucose by the process known as glycogenolysis. Homeostasis of blood glucose is maintained by the hormones insulin and glucagon secreted by the pancreas. Glycogen from the liver supplies glucose to all tissues in the horse's body including the brain, nerve and blood cells. Glycogen stored in the muscles, however, is for muscle use only.

Approximately 95% of glycogen is stored in the horse's muscles. Greater muscle mass may be produced through work and will increase the amount of glycogen that can be stored by the horse. Glucose may also be formed by the horse's body cells from non-carbohydrate substances including amino acids, lactate, pyruvate and glycerol. This process is known as gluconeogenesis. All non-essential amino acids and some essential amino acids are glucogenic, which means the carbon skeleton may be used to produce glucose.

## Adenosine triphosphate (ATP)

The main source of readily available energy in the horse's cells is ATP or adenosine triphosphate. ATP is generated from the metabolism of energy giving substrates as mentioned previously including carbohydrates, fats and proteins with glucose being the main source of carbohydrate for energy production.

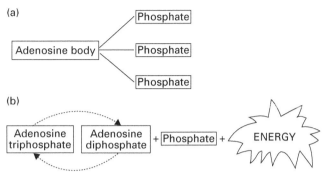

**Figure 6.4**  Structure of ATP.

Energy is actually produced from the splitting of a chemical bond in the ATP molecule within the horse's cells. ATP is often termed the cells' energy currency. ATP consists of an adenosine body with three phosphate groups attached (Figure 6.4a and b).

Energy is released from the removal of one of these three phosphate groups resulting in ADP (adenosine diphosphate)

$$ATP \rightarrow ADP + P + Energy\ release\ (8\,kcal/mole)$$

This chemical process also results in the loss of roughly 75% of the energy by the production of heat, which is why horses become hot and sweaty when working. Once the ATP has been 'used' and converted to ADP, the ADP must be converted back into ATP by using the energy produced from food. This adds the third phosphorus to ADP in a process known as oxidative phosphorylation which is the driving force for many biochemical reactions within the horse's body including nutrient absorption from the digestive tract.

Chemical breakdown of 1 mole of glucose by glycolysis in the presence of oxygen results in 38 molecules of ATP, whereas in the absence of oxygen this is two molecules ATP (Figure 6.5a and b). The body stores only small amounts of ATP at any one time – just sufficient to maintain basic living requirements at rest. When the horse starts to move or exercise, energy demand increases and the supply of ATP is rapidly used up.

## Energy measurement

Energy is ultimately given off from the horse's body as heat therefore energy is measured in units of heat or joules.

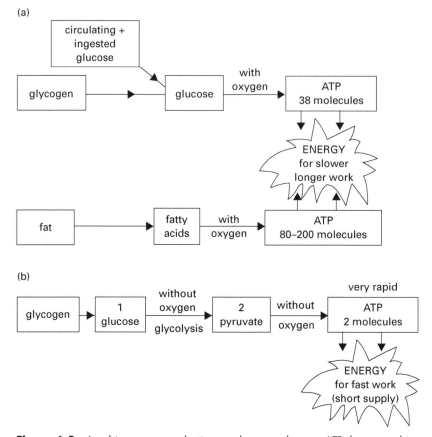

**Figure 6.5**   Aerobic energy production produces much more ATP than anerobic.

*1 Joule is the energy required to move a weight of 1 kilogram over a distance of 1 metre, by a force of 1 Newton.*

However the imperial units of heat or calories are still widely used particularly in the USA.

*1 calorie is defined as the amount of heat required to increase the temperature of 1 gram of water by 1 degree centigrade.*

In reality both the calorie and joule are very small and so megacalories (1 Mcal = 1000 kilocalories) or megajoules (1 MJ = 1000 kilojoules) are normally used for horses.

- Mcal – used in the USA for horses
- MJ – used in the UK for horses.

To convert megacalories to megajoules simply multiply by 4.184 (4.2)

1 Mcal = 4.184 or 4.2 MJ

100 Mcal = 418.4 or 420 MJ

To convert megajoules to megacalories simply divide by 4.184 or 4.2

500 MJ/4.184 = 119.5 or 120 Mcal

In human nutrition energy is generally measured as kilocalories (kcal) but actually described as calories. A human energy requirement of 2000 'calories' per day is actually 2000 kcal or 2.0 Mcal, which is 8.37 MJ. This can be quite confusing.

# Energy for work

The horse's body has three main energy systems it can call upon for physical work:

- ATP-PC or phosphagen system
- Aerobic system
- Anaerobic system.

As mentioned previously little ATP is stored and so when the horse begins working, ATP has to be produced from one of these three energy producing systems from three different biochemical pathways. The rate of ATP production from each of the three systems is very different and which one or which combination is used depends upon the level of exercise and supply of oxygen into the body cells from respiration in the lungs.

## ATP-PC system

This is the ATP-phosphocreatine pathway and results in an immediate release of energy as required for short sprints or maximal bursts of speed for up to approximately 6 seconds. Muscles use stored ATP or CP (PCr /phosphocreatine), which has been derived from glucose or free fatty acids, as an immediate source of energy. Phosphocreatine is another high energy compound similar to ATP, formed by linking a phosphate molecule to a protein known as creatine. Creatine is a protein made from three amino acids (arginine, lysine and glycine) mainly in the liver. Creatine is then taken from the liver to body cells where it is used to make phosphocreatine. Once phosphocreatine has been used for energy it is either recycled or excreted from the kidneys as creatine.

The ATP-PC system involves phosphocreatine losing its phosphate and transferring it to ADP to make ATP (Figure 6.6) In addition, an

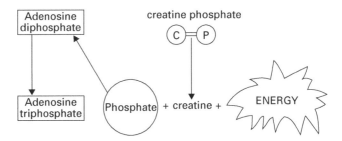

**Figure 6.6**  The ATP-PC system.

immediate and short supply of energy may be fuelled by glycolysis in muscle cells, which converts glucose to pyruvate in the absence of oxygen, i.e. under anaerobic conditions. This provides enough energy for a short sprint or for a short time at maximal speed, i.e. only a matter of minutes. If further energy is required then the complete breakdown of pyruvate (and fatty acids) via the TCA cycle in the mitochondria is required and this needs oxygen.

### Aerobic system

Aerobic simply means requiring 'air' or oxygen. Aerobic exercise tends to be slower and of longer duration. This allows time for the transport of sufficient amounts of oxygen from the lungs to muscles and for glucose to generate ATP from glycolysis, i.e. the breakdown of carbohydrates and fat in the presence of oxygen. Under these circumstances 38 molecules of ATP are produced which is approximately 20 times more efficient than the anaerobic energy system. Production of ATP through the aerobic system is slower than the ATP-PC system or anaerobic system, but produces much more ATP. The aerobic system will kick in during slower exercise after a very short time and will continue to supply energy over a much longer time. Most of the carbohydrate immediately comes from the breakdown of stored muscle glycogen and then additional glucose from the bloodstream is used as muscle glycogen supplies run out and exercise continues. For endurance horses this carbohydrate may be supplied by food consumed during the ride. Fatty acids may also be used but can only be used in the presence of oxygen, i.e. only under aerobic conditions. Fatty acids supply even greater amounts of energy, i.e. one fatty acid may produce as much as 80-200 molecules of ATP depending upon its type (see Figure 6.5). During aerobic exercise the choice of fatty acids or glucose varies according to several factors namely:

- Duration of exercise
- Intensity of exercise
- Fitness level of the horse
- Horse's diet.

During aerobic exercise, a mixture of fats and glycogen is used. As exercise speed increases so does the horse's reliance and use of muscle glycogen. For slow speeds such as walking and trotting in endurance type exercise, exercise is fuelled mainly from fatty acids and this is why fat is a very useful food energy source for endurance and long distance equine activities.

As glycogen becomes depleted, blood glucose is used which eventually will run out if further glucose is not made available from food or gluconeogenesis.

## Anaerobic system

Anaerobic exercise takes place in the absence of 'air' or oxygen. This system kicks in as soon as high intensity work begins such as in a sprint race. This is the dominant energy source for fats work up to approximately 90 seconds. In order to meet this sudden huge energy requirement, glucose bypasses the normal aerobic energy system and follows a different route, namely glycogen. Muscle glycogen is broken down to glucose as described previously and undergoes glycolysis resulting in pyruvate. Pyruvate in the absence of oxygen is broken down to lactate (lactic acid) releasing ATP, instead of entering the TCA cycle in the mitochondria. This process results in only 2 ATP molecules per glucose molecule, which is highly inefficient. Although this process is rapid, it also results in the build-up of lactic acid in the muscle cells resulting in the onset of fatigue and the muscles can no longer contract. The horse has to slow down or stop to recover. Once this happens oxygen becomes available again and the lactate is used in one of two ways (Figure 6.7):

- Converted back to pyruvate in the presence of oxygen and then enters the TCA cycle to form ATP (i.e. the aerobic system)
- Transported via the blood and converted to glucose in the liver via gluconeogenesis for immediate use or stored as glycogen.

Lactic acid is therefore a valuable fuel (not a waste product) after the initial high intensity exercise is reduced. Lactic acid is usually cleared from the muscle cells quite rapidly following intensive exercise and may be recycled as soon as 15 minutes afterwards.

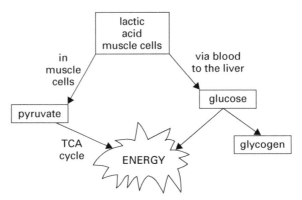

**Figure 6.7** Fate of lactate following exercise.

## Types of muscle fibre

There are several different types of muscle fibre within each muscle in horses and this is exactly the same as in humans. They are broadly grouped into fast twitch (FT) or Type II for fast contraction or slow twitch (ST) or Type I for slower endurance type work. Both fast twitch and slow twitch muscle fibres use all three energy systems to produce ATP, however the FT fibres use mainly the anaerobic glycolytic systems as mentioned above or the ATP-PC rapid system. The ST fibres use mainly the aerobic system for endurance type work and are also known as ST high oxidative fibres.

The FT fibres are categorised by having a high glycolytic activity. These are further subdivided into FT high oxidative and FT low oxidative fibres.

Horses are born with a specific distribution of muscle fibre types and the proportion of FT and ST muscle fibres can vary among individual horses. The quarter horse, for example, has a higher number of FT muscle fibre types than the Arab, which is better suited to endurance. FT fibres have a greater diameter in order to generate more power, which results in a bulkier physique as seen in sprint horses. However, some adaptations in total muscle fibre types occur during training. Endurance work needs more muscle fibres that can contract relatively slowly for longer times, i.e. they are more resistant to fatigue. Sprinters require more fast contracting fibres that unfortunately are prone to rapid fatigue.

Slow twitch muscle fibres have a higher propensity to use oxygen, which means they can keep contracting for longer at a slower rate.

## Partition of food energy

The energy of a feedstuff can be burnt in a bomb calorimeter in the presence of oxygen to measure its gross energy (GE). However this GE is not all available to the horse as there are losses in the body. Some energy escapes via the digestive tract as faeces. The resulting energy is known as digestible energy (DE). Further energy is lost via urine and from gases produced by the digestive system and this leaves metabolisable energy (ME). Further energy is lost as heat and this leaves the net energy (NE) (Figure 6.8).

In the UK and USA, the energy in a feedstuff is usually given in terms of digestible energy (DE) in MJ/kg. These are given as dry matter values (DM). The apparent DE of a feed is calculated by subtracting the gross energy in the faeces from the gross energy in the feed ingested. This is apparent because some energy also comes not just from the feed but also from cells sloughed off the inside of the digestive tract and also from digestive secretions.

Digestible energy can be determined by one of three methods:

- Feeding trials
- Chemical analysis and predictive equations
- Data table that lists DE values.

Feeding trials are the most accurate way of determining DE measurements of feeds, but these are very expensive.

Previously DE values were estimated from scientific data acquired from other agricultural animals such as pigs and sheep. This was not ideal. DE for horses is therefore calculated by predictive equations developed by the NRC from known analysed chemical composition of feeds such as those shown below.

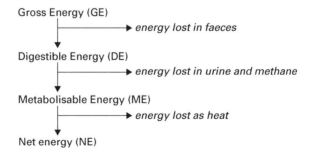

**Figure 6.8** Partition of food energy.

### NRC 1989 equations

1) To estimate DE for dry forage, fresh forage and pasture

$$DE\,(Mcal/kg) = 4.22 - 0.11 \times (\%ADF) + 0.0332 \times (\%CP) + 0.00112 \times (\%ADF^2)$$

2) To estimate DE for energy feeds and protein supplements

$$DE(Mcal/kg) = 4.07 - 0.055 \times (\%ADF)$$

where ADF is acid detergent fibre and CP is srude protein.

Using further data from Pagan, another equation was later used from 1998.

### Pagan 1998 equation

$$DE(Kcal/kg) = 2118 + 12.18 \times (\%CP) - 9.37 \times (\%ADF) - 3.83 \times (\%hemicellulose) + 47.18 \times (\%fat) + 20.35 \times (\% \text{ non-structural CHO}) - 26.3(\%ash)$$

Hemicellulose is determined from (ADF – NDF and non-structural CHO).

Non-structural CHO = 100 – %NDF – %Fat – %Ash – %CP.

Unfortunately neither of these equations was considered accurate enough for feedstuffs high in fat and also those high in fibre.

Zeyner and Kienzle therefore developed a further equation in 2002.

### Zeyner & Kienzle 2002 equation

$$DE\ MJ/Kg\ DM = -3.6 + 0.211 \times (\%CP) + 0.421 \times (\%AEE) + 0.015 \times (\%CF) + 0.189 \times (\%NFE)$$

AEE is acid ether extract, CF is crude fibre and NFE is nitrogen free extract.

In reality the NRC 1989 DE equation works well for cereals, cereal by-products and other by-product feeds such as beet pulp. The Zeyner calculation would appear to be more useful for high fat feeds.

Equations can be used therefore to estimated DE of feedstuffs. Alternatively there are tables that give DE values such as can be found in NRC *Nutrient Requirements of Horses* 6th edition. This is a much simpler method for the average horse owner.

## Net energy

The NE or Net Energy system was introduced in France in 1984 by INRA. This was further updated in 1990. This system begins with ME whereby the metabolisable energy may be transformed to Recovered Energy (RE) or to heat. The heat energy (HE) is the total Heat Energy lost to the environment.

HE components include:

- Basal metabolism
- Voluntary activity
- Thermal regulation
- Product formation, e.g. milk, foetus, etc.
- Digestion and absorption
- Waste formation and excretion
- Fermentation.

The NE system provides the NE content of feedstuffs for maintenance first. The feed values in this scheme are expressed as UFCs (*Unite Fourragere Cheval* or more simply horse feed units).

The NE system uses barley as a reference value of 1.

1 kg barley = 1 UFC = 9.414 MJ/NE

The UFC for maize for example is 1.33 MJ/NE

The DE system gives the following

Barley DE = 15.2 MJ/kg
Maize DE = 16.1 MJ/kg

The NE system uses the following information:

- Data from GE and digestibility values of feedstuffs
- Efficiency of conversion of DE to ME in horses
- Proportion of energy supplied by absorbed nutrients
- Efficiency of ME utilisation of absorbed nutrients.

Although more accurate theoretically than the DE system, the NE system is deemed too difficult for routine use. The complexity of the NE system is a major disadvantage over the NRC's DE system. Another disadvantage is the use of barley as a reference point given that may horse feeders do not feed barley.

The NE system has been accepted very well for other species of livestock and is used more widely for cattle in the USA. However, the DE system is still preferred by the majority of equine nutritionists, feed manufacturers and vets in both the UK and USA.

**Summary points**

- Energy is not a nutrient, but supplies fuel for life.
- Energy is chemically derived from nutrients such as carbohydrates (soluble and insoluble), i.e. including fibre, lipids/fats and amino acids.
- Horses undergoing very fast work for short speeds use energy differently from horses doing slower work over long periods such as endurance.
- Fat is the most concentrated source of energy providing the horse's body with almost twice as much energy as carbohydrates or protein.
- Red blood cells and brain cells depend almost entirely upon glucose as an energy source.
- The horse's body has three main energy systems it can call upon for physical work, ATP-PC system, aerobic system, anaerobic system.
- Megacalories (1 Mcal = 1000 kilocalories) or megajoules (1 MJ = 1000 kilojoules) is normally used for horses.
- Glycogen storage within the horse's body is limited.
- Glucose may also be formed from non-carbohydrate substances including amino acids, lactate, pyruvate and glycerol.
- The horse's body stores only small amounts of ATP at any one time just sufficient to maintain its basic living requirements at rest.
- During aerobic exercise, a mixture of fats and glycogen is used.
- Lactic acid is a highly valuable fuel after the initial high intensity exercised is reduced.
- The build-up of lactic acid in the muscle cells resulting in the onset of fatigue.
- The DE system for calculating energy in feedstuffs is preferred to the NE system and is therefore much more widely used.

# Forage for Horses

Forage is the main feed for all herbivores, including horses, providing food for the majority of horses all year round. Conserved (harvested and stored) forage such as hay, haylage and chaffs (including straw) provide valuable nutrients and energy for horses from plant sources. Horses rely upon the fermentation of insoluble carbohydrate (fibre) in the hindgut for their main energy supply. The protein, vitamin and mineral content of forage is highly variable. Legumes such as alfalfa contain higher amounts of protein, calcium and magnesium for example. Straw is very low in protein and higher in indigestible fibre.

Forage can therefore range from lush spring grass to straw. Mineral content (particularly trace minerals) varies tremendously according to soil, area, plant species and fertilisation. Sodium levels also vary from very low to high. Pastures in the UK unless extremely acidic or wet are unlikely to be deficient in calcium, phosphorus, potassium or magnesium, however trace minerals are more likely to be deficient particularly in some areas. Copper, selenium and zinc are commonly low.

Pasture provides fluctuating energy almost on a daily basis and so makes it difficult to assess accurately for the purposes of formulating rations. According to NRC *Nutrient Requirements of Horses* 6th revised edition, a 500 kg mature horse will voluntarily consume approximately 9–10 kg dry matter of pasture per day. Protein levels are generally good in pasture and are much higher in spring with young grasses growing at a fast rate. Protein and overall pasture digestibility falls over the season with a small increase in autumn, whereas fibre increases. Vitamin levels are high in growing pasture but fall when grass becomes dormant over winter.

The main factor determining the nutritive value of forage is the stage of maturity at grazing or harvest (Table 7.1).

Crude protein in particular declines rapidly through the growing season, as does soluble carbohydrate, whereas lignin and crude fibre

**Table 7.1**   Table showing the effect of the stage of maturity of orchard grass.

|  | Early pasture | Early hay | Late hay |
|---|---|---|---|
| Crude protein % | 24.8 | 13.0 | 12.4 |
| Sugars % | 2.1 | 0.8 | 0.9 |
| Lignin % | 5.7 | 6.2 | 8.1 |
| Crude fibre % | 26.9 | 31.8 | 35.0 |

increase. Digestibility of pasture also falls. These changes will depend upon the weather during the growing season and the application of fertilisers but these factors have relatively little impact compared with the stage of maturity shown above.

Harvest and storage methods also affect the nutritive value of forage, for example hay or haylage cut later in the year usually contain fewer nutrients.

## PASTURE

For horses, herbage is often divided into native and cultivated species of grasses belong to the family *Gramineae* and some of the most common are shown in Figure 7.1; they may be divided into the following:

• Cool season grasses – e.g. Kentucky blue grass, tall fescue, perennial ryegrass, Italian ryegrass, timothy, meadow fescue
• Warm season grasses – e.g. Bermuda grass
• Legumes – e.g. alfalfa, white clover, red clover.

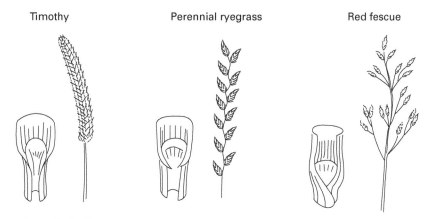

**Figure 7.1**   Some common pasture grasses.

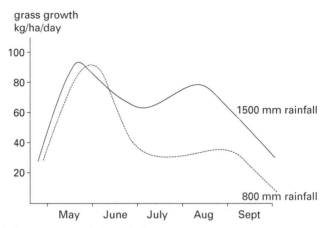

grass growth
kg/ha/day

1500 mm rainfall

800 mm rainfall

May    June    July    Aug    Sept

**Figure 7.2**  Grass growth through the season.

Cool season grasses generally mature at slower rates than warm season grasses. Cool season grasses start to grow at 7 degrees Celsius (°C) with optimum growth between 16 °C and 24 °Cwhereas warm season grasses start growing at 15 °C with an optimal temperature for growth of 32–35 °C. Grass growth throughout the season is shown in Figure 7.2 (temperate regions such as UK).

Pasture may at certain times of the year not supply enough energy such as over winter and horses need to be supplemented with conserved forage and additional concentrates if required. In the spring and summer, pasture may supply too much energy resulting in very overweight horses and ponies and a higher risk of laminitis. Spring pasture is often low in dry matter (containing high levels of water) and grazing horses often crave high dry matter forage such as hay. Horses may be seen licking soil or chewing wood during the early spring. In early spring it is therefore a good idea to put hay out to ensure adequate dry matter and fibre intake.

High quality, permanent pasture not only provides an excellent and natural source of food, but also a safe turnout and exercise area (Figure 7.3). Permanent pasture includes a combination of plants including grasses, clover, herbs and often weeds. Grassland comprises a large percentage of agricultural land, particularly in the UK and USA.

Permanent pasture consists of grass that has grown naturally over many years. It contains a much wider variety of grasses and plants. When young grasses are sown, they grow upright, leaving patches of soil between them. These are soon filled by native grasses providing a carpet otherwise known as the 'sward'. This carpeting is more able to

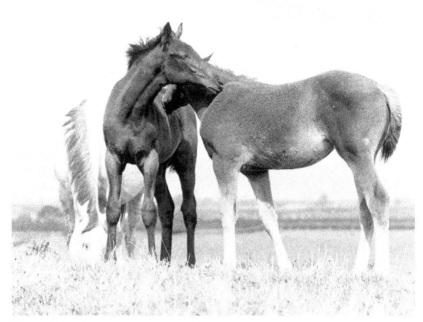

**Figure 7.3**  Good pasture also provides a safe turn out area for exercise. (Courtesy of Jo Prestwich)

withstand grazing by horses and reduces the likelihood of poaching, particularly in the winter months.

Rough grazing normally refers to moorland and hills and has to be tough to survive the harsh weather conditions. These conditions may be suitable for hardy ponies and overweight types.

Unfortunately, grass does not grow in an even pattern throughout the year. In addition, pasture varies tremendously in nutrient content over the season (Figure 7.4). There are many factors affecting grass growth, including temperature, soil, rainfall, stocking rates, fertilisation, topping, poaching, etc.

Most grasses grow as single plants and spread outwards by the growth of new shoots called tillers. Each tiller produces both roots and leaves and consequently they grow their own branching root systems. Some types of grass can spread across the ground by creeping stems just above or below the surface (Figure 7.5).

Normally growth begins in earnest in spring when the soil warms up. The growing point of the plant is at ground level, at the centre of the plant, and is therefore protected to some degree.

When stocking rates are too high, horses graze closer to the ground and remove these vital growing points. However, some removal of the

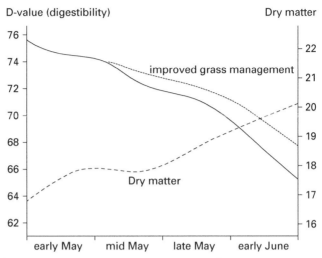

**Figure 7.4**  Pasture varies in nutrient content over the season.

leaves (defoliation) stimulates the growth of the grass plant and there-fore the sward. If the leaves are not removed by grazing or topping, i.e. the mechanical cutting of the sward, then the plant will continue to grow through its natural life cycle and flower.

Overgrazing will result in too few leaves available to photosynthe-sise and produce energy for further new leaf growth thus reducing overall growth rate of the pasture.

Flowering or 'heading' involves the development of tillers into upright fibrous stalks, which produce flowers and then seeds. After dispersal of the seeds many of the leaves wither and die, leaving fibrous stalks, i.e. the pasture becomes nutritionally poor. These fibrous stalks contain a woody material known as lignin, which enables the grass plant to physically support the flower head and seeds. Horses are unable to digest lignin and intake of large amounts of this woody type material may give horses, particularly youngstock, a 'hay belly', and reduce voluntary intake of food.

Young spring grass contains very few woody stems and is of good nutritional quality, containing high levels of water, protein and soluble carbohydrates (sugars).

## Clover (*Trifolium* sp.)

Clover is a legume often seen in temperate horse pastures (Figure 7.6). Legumes have root nodules where nitrogen fixing takes place. The

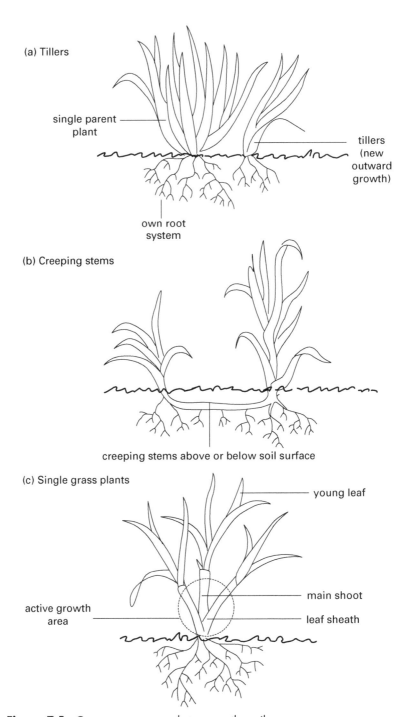

(a) Tillers

single parent plant

own root system

tillers (new outward growth)

(b) Creeping stems

creeping stems above or below soil surface

(c) Single grass plants

young leaf

main shoot

leaf sheath

active growth area

**Figure 7.5**   Grass grows outwards to cover the soil.

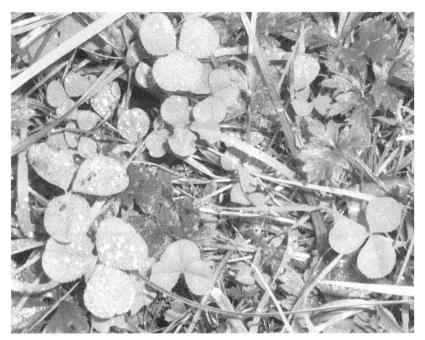

**Figure 7.6** Clover.

most common clovers are red and white clover. Clovers are nutrition-ally superior to grass, containing higher protein levels and also miner-als including calcium, phosphorus, magnesium and copper. Sugar levels in clover are similar to grasses and, although clovers do not generally contain much fructan, they do contain starch, levels of which may be quite high particularly in red clover.

## Lawn clippings

These are unacceptable as a feed for horses under any circumstances. The small particle size and high moisture content of grass cut with a mower results in rapid fermentation in warm weather. Feeding lawn clippings and other garden waste such as potatoes, tomatoes and rhubarb to horses can lead to colic, botulism, laminitis and may even be fatal and so should be avoided.

## Conserved forage

The main principle for conserving forage (usually grass) for future feeding to horses is to reduce moisture content and/or oxygen to stop the natural decay that normally begins following mowing in the field. When making hay the water content of the hay crop must be reduced from 65–85% to 20% or less over three to five days. This is achieved by sun drying in the field or air/heat drying in a barn for barn dried hay. Haylage, on the other hand, is wilted to a water content of 45–50%, before being wrapped to enable 'pickling' of the crop in an oxygen free environment, this is known as ensiling. Haylage therefore does not need as much drying time. When haylage was first made for horses, it was cut earlier in the year when grass is lush, higher in protein and energy and lower in fibre, perhaps too much for most horses. Today haylage for horses tends to be cut later as the end product is more suitable. Hay contains less water than haylage which in turn contains less water than silage (Figure 7.7).

## Hay

This is the most traditional method of conserving grass. It can vary tremendously in nutritional content, mostly determined by the time of year it is harvested; this in turn is often predetermined by the weather. In some years, owing to high rainfall, hay is not harvested early in the year but left until later even as long as September and this hay will be of poor nutritional value.

There are two types of hay, namely meadow hay and seed hay. Meadow hay contains many different grass and herb species, all maturing at different times through the summer. This results in more leaf and seed heads and is normally less stalky and softer to touch. Seed hay is now thought to be single species grass hay such as Ryegrass or

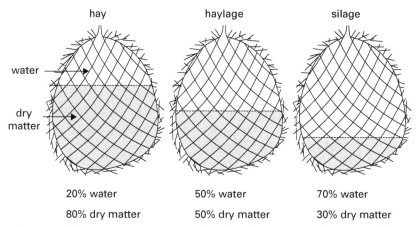

**Figure 7.7** Diagrammatic representation of moisture content of conserved forage.

Timothy. This is generally stalkier and less leafy than meadow hay and so feels harder to the touch than meadow hay. Seed hay is often lower in protein than meadow hay.

Hay tends to be less nutritious than haylage as it is cut later (Figure 7.8), however this is not always the case. Hay usually contains medium protein and low to average sugars with good levels of digestible fibre to maintain gut health and function.

Good hay will have been cut and dried thoroughly at the right time, baled and stored properly. The problem with hay tends to be related to its hygienic quality. The weather conditions are not always favourable for thorough drying and mown hay is often rained upon. Barn dried hay however relies less upon the weather.

There is some confusion about dust in hay; in fact it may come from one of three different sources:

• Moulds and fungi may grow on cut hay prior to baling in damp weather conditions or may grow on baled hay at higher temperatures when hay has been baled too damp

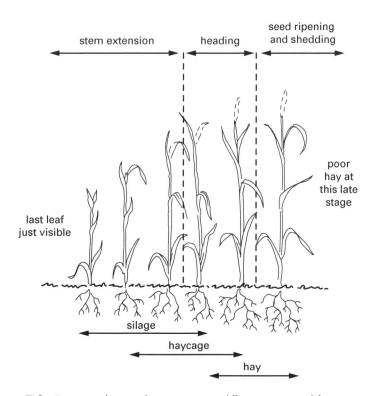

**Figure 7.8** Diagram showing best time to cut different conserved forage.

- Soil splash from previous heavy rain
- Leaf shatter resulting from very dry hay-leaves breaking and shattering during baling.

Dust containing moulds and fungi can result in respiratory disease such as COPD (chronic obstructive pulmonary disease) in horses (Figure 7.9).

The quantity and quality of field dried hay for harvesting will depend upon several factors including:

- Stage of maturity when cut
- Methods of handling
- Moisture content
- Weather conditions during drying, has it been rained upon, for example.

Rain falling on very newly cut hay will do far less damage than rain falling on hay that is partially dried. Rapid drying results in the fewest changes to the nutritive value of the hay crop. Hay stored in the barn when too damp may undergo fermentation, which results in heating and occasionally spontaneous combustion. The heated hay gives rise to thermophilic mould growth, which is very undesirable.

Hay that has been made properly does not need to be stored in the barn before feeding, it can be fed straight away while it is still relatively nutritious; however, hay is mostly stored for a month or two before

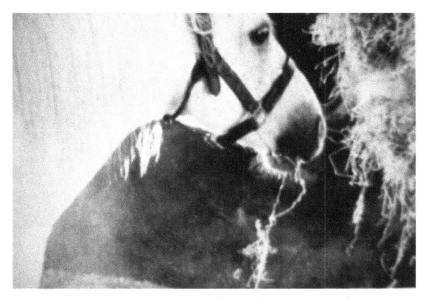

**Figure 7.9** 'Dust' in hay may cause and exascerbate respiratory disease.

use. Feeding one-year-old hay that has been left to gather dust in a barn and which has lost all its vitamins is not ideal. Hay may be soaked to reduce dust levels and to swell any fungal spores that may be present to a size where they should become harmless. Soaked hay should be fully submerged in water for 20 to 30 minutes and no longer prior to feeding. However, for horses and ponies prone to laminitis it can be soaked for an hour maximum to help remove any soluble sugars present. When feeding new hay, it should be introduced slowly.

## Haylage

The making of haylage is probably more suited to the weather in the UK. Haylage is grass that has been preserved by ensiling. The grass crop is usually cut slightly earlier than hay and wilted to moisture content of about 45–50%. This is then wrapped tightly in bales to exclude oxygen (Figure 7.10). A fermentation process then takes place and increasing acidity from the pickling process drops the pH to about 5.0. At this pH, moulds and fungi cannot grow and at the end of the fermentation process the haylage will remain stable as long as the bag or wrapping remains fully intact. This can take up to 8–10 weeks. Making good haylage requires farming expertise and if grass is ensiled when it is too dry or it doesn't contain enough soluble sugars,

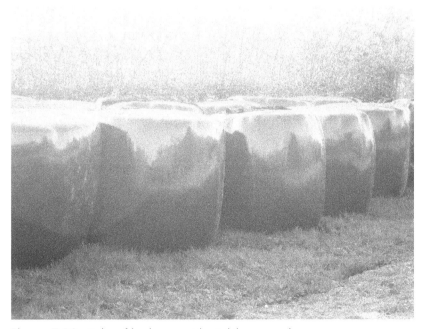

**Figure 7.10**  Bales of haylage must be tightly wrapped.

incomplete fermentation occurs. In these cases, pH levels do not fall low enough as there is not enough acid produced by the fermentation process and there is a greater growth of undesirable moulds and fungi. Haylage that has undergone incomplete fermentation or that has undergone secondary fermentation/heating can be a health hazard to horses. In addition this can result in the production of ammonia, which may irritate the horse's airways – a particular problem for working horses.

Botulism is a concern when feeding haylage and the *Clostridium botulinum* organism tends to proliferate in very wet haylage. Clostridia are bacteria that live in the soil and may contaminate the haylage crop via close cutting, from mud splashing or from deceased animals. However, haylage with a dry matter above 50% is too dry for clostridia to multiply. Outbreaks of botulism poisoning from haylage are not uncommon and vaccination is becoming more available. Where botulism has been a problem, vaccinations should be discussed with the vet.

There are eight toxin types produced by different strains of bacteria namely A, B, C1, C2, D, E, F and G. Type 6 accounts for more than 80% of equine botulism cases.

Yeasts may grow on haylage cut with high levels of soluble sugars and although small amounts of white spots are not harmful too much yeast can cause aerobic instability of the haylage.

Feeding too little haylage is common. Haylage contains more water than hay and so more haylage needs to be fed than hay to ensure the dry matter intake is adequate. For example if haylage contains one-third more water than hay, then one-third more haylage should be fed, to ensure DM intake. Feeding small daily amounts in small nets is not recommended under any circumstances. When assessing the costs, it is important to remember that haylage is heavier than hay as it contains more water.

The following parameters show haylage has fermented and is safe to feed. The supplier of haylage should provide a basic analysis prior to purchase.

Good haylage contains:

- Dry matter, 55–70%
- PH. 5.0–6.0
- Ammonia N less than 5.0%
- Ash, less than 8% (high ash may indicate presence of soil and more undesirable microorganisms)
- Crude protein, 7–12%
- MAD fibre, 32–38%.

## Choosing hay or haylage

The choice of hay or haylage often depends upon local availability, the number of horses and size of the bales. Well made, good quality hay is probably safer to feed to most horses and ponies, particularly if it is soaked. Haylage is preferred for horses in hard work or with known respiratory conditions, but it must have fermented thoroughly and been made specifically for horses i.e. not too high in protein and with adequate fibre.

Haylage tends to contain higher levels of energy and protein and so fewer concentrates may be required. However, it must be used within 3–5 days once opened as it will deteriorate on exposure to air. Any haylage that appears to smell 'off' or is discoloured should be returned to the supplier and should not be fed. Furthermore, mouldy hay or haylage should never be fed to horses under any circumstances.

## Straw and chaff

There are many different chaff products available for horses. Straw consists of the stems with some leaves after the removal of grains. Straw is more stalky and fibrous than hay with very little leaf (Figure 7.11a and b). The most common straw chaffs are wheat, barley and oat straw. Straw chaffs are very low in protein, low in digestibility, very high in fibre and often high in lignin, which horses cannot digest, i.e. they are of poor feeding value. However, straw chaffs can be useful for very overweight horses and ponies.

Straw may also be contaminated with mycotoxins produced by different fungi. During wet weather, *Fusarium*, a saprophytic fungus, may invade the heads of grain. *Fusarium* can produce a number of mycotoxins that are poisonous to horses.

Straw is more useful when mixed with other dried chopped forage such as hay or alfalfa and should only be fed to horses with good dentition.

Other chaffs include dried grass alfalfa mixes, meadow hay or seed hay mixes. Alfalfa is highly nutritious as is chopped dried grass. Chaffs may be molassed or contain dried fruit such as apple. Some chaffs contain additional oil for energy and coat condition. They may also be fortified with vitamins and minerals to make a complete feed.

## Dried grass chaff

Dried grass is sometimes cut and turned into a chaff product. The grass is harvested at a highly nutritious stage of growth and then rapidly

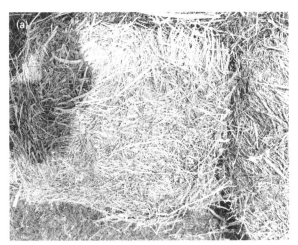

**Figure 7.11a** Hay contains more leaf.

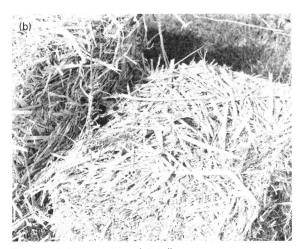

**Figure 7.11b** Straw contains more 'woody' stalk.

dried at high temperatures of up to 800 °C within a few hours of leaving the field. This ensures any moulds or spores are killed. Dried grass therefore has a feed value virtually identical to fresh grass without the water so care should be taken when feeding. Dried grass contains high levels of digestible fibre and important antioxidants including vitamin E and beta-carotene, and a correct calcium/phosphorus ratio, generally.

## Alfalfa/lucerne

Alfalfa is from the legume family or *Leguminosae* which includes alfalfa and clover (*Trifolium* sp.) see earlier. Alfalfa is commonly grown as a

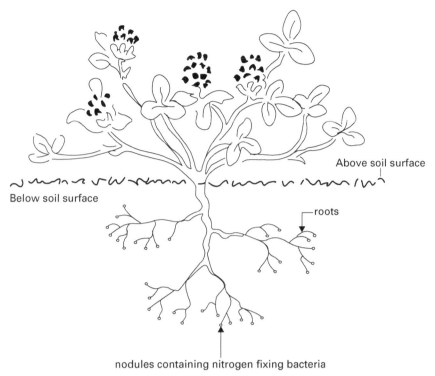

Below soil surface

Above soil surface

roots

nodules containing nitrogen fixing bacteria

**Figure 7.12** Nodules of legumes including alfalfa and clover contain nitrogen fixing bacteria.

crop for harvesting in the UK as it tends to be cut and dried and/or chopped for feeding. In the USA alfalfa is often used for grazing and/ or hay. Alfalfa, although high in protein, can also contain high levels of digestible fibre owing to the more fibrous stem. Alfalfa chaffs are nutritious having been cut at the optimum time and rapidly dried at very high temperatures maintaining the nutritional value. Sometimes, once bagged and stored, leaf shatter may result in a dark coloured dust. The stem, which looks like straw may be quite hard for same horses. This may occur even though molasses or oil may have been added to the chaff. This should be taken into account for horses with poor dentition, for example.

Legumes are able to fix atmospheric nitrogen, because of their symbiotic relationship with certain bacteria found in the root nodules of these plants (Figure 7.12). They therefore tend to be higher in protein. Alfalfa also contains lower levels of soluble carbohydrates (unlike spring grass) and is often used to feed horses requiring low sugar/ starch diets such as laminitics and those that tie up.

Recent research suggests that alfalfa may also help reduce the severity of gastric ulcers but it is not a replacement for omeprazole and other veterinary treatments.

## Grass nuts/cubes

Grass and alfalfa are often cut at an early growth stage and then dried with a dry matter content of roughly 88%. In the UK the crude protein must be at least 13%. High protein grass pellets must contain at least 16% crude protein (CP), whereas dried alfalfa contains 15–20% CP.

These products contain high levels of important antioxidant vitamins, such as vitamin E and beta-carotene. Grass pellets are often included in coarse mixes and other compound feeds. They may also be fed as a single ingredient feed, but should be analyzed to check for possible mineral imbalances/deficiencies.

---

**Sumary points**

- Forage is the main feed for all horses.
- Fibre is not a filler for horses – it provides energy.
- Nutrient content of forage is highly variable.
- Hay tends to be less nutritious than haylage as it is cut later.
- Dust containing moulds and fungi can result in respiratory disease such as COPD in horses.
- Haylage is preferred for horses in hard work or with known respiratory conditions.
- Botulism is a concern when feeding haylage and tends to be a problem in wet haylage.
- Straw may be contaminated with mycotoxins produced by different fungi.

# Feedstuffs

Feedstuffs provide the raw materials for horse feeds. An understanding of the most common feedstuffs and the nutrients they supply to horses is vital when working out rations for all types of horses. Factors which may affect the acceptability of a feedstuff for horses include cost, palatability, digestibility and availability of nutrients within it.

A feedstuff may be defined as any component of the horse's diet that serves some useful function. Most feedstuffs for horses provide several nutrients:

- Forage – wet or dry (Chapter 7)
- Energy concentrates – cereals, milling by-products, molasses, beet pulp, fats (mainly vegetable), rice bran, brewery by-products
- Protein concentrates, oilseed meals (soybean, linseed, sunflower), marine meals, dehydrated legumes, single cell sources, e.g. yeast
- Chaff based products with/without added cereals and/or premix
- Mineral supplements
- Vitamin supplements
- Non-nutritive additives, e.g. , buffers, flavours, enzymes, mycotoxin binders, yeasts, miscellaneous.

## CONCENTRATES

Concentrates are fed to increase energy supply or energy density. High energy feedstuffs include cereal grains and cereal by-products. Liquid feeds such as molasses and oils are also included as concentrates. Energy from concentrate feedstuffs is supplied primarily by soluble carbohydrates (sugars and starch) or by fats/lipids.

When forage alone is not enough to meet horses' energy requirements, for example working horses and fast growing/lactating breeding stock, concentrates may need to be fed. Traditionally horses have been fed cereals as an energy source. Oats have been the cereal of choice for many years, particularly for working and breeding horses e.g. racehorses in training. Many studs have grown their own oats and some farm-based studs still do. However, cereals are not a natural feed for horses. The digestive tract of the horse is suited more to a forage diet. Cereals should therefore always be fed with care, and little and often.

# CEREAL GRAINS

Cereal grains are the seeds of plants such as oats, barley, maize (corn) and wheat. These are in fact members of the grass family (*Graminae*). In some equestrian circles all cereals and compound feeds are grouped together under the general heading 'corn' but in the USA corn refers specifically to maize. Leading to more confusion, in the UK each of the cereals is commonly referred to as 'straights'.

Cereal grains are less variable in nutritive quality than forage, but they are commonly low in calcium and sodium. The carbohydrates in cereal grains are mainly starch with small amounts of sugars. Starches from the various cereal grains have different physical characteristics when viewed under a microscope and the size of the starch granules contained within the endosperm varies. Some small differences can be seen in the ratio of amylose to amylopectin for example (see Chapter 3). Amylose is a long straight molecule, which is less easy to digest enzymically than amylopectin, which consists of branched chains. The more amylose the cereal contains the slower it is generally digested, i.e. lower GI (glycaemic index) – see below.

Cereals also contain low levels of essential amino acids, i.e. protein quality is relatively poor. In addition all cereals have reverse calcium to phosphorus ratio, which means they contain much more phosphorus than calcium, the opposite of the horses requirements.

The high starch content of cereal grains means that great care should be taken when feeding them. If large amounts are fed at any one feed there is a higher risk of undigested starch passing through the foregut without being digested and swamping the hindgut where it is rapidly fermented by the hindgut microbes. This may further lead to hindgut acidosis, laminitis, colic and diarrhoea. The maximum amount of cereal straights or high starch compound feeds to give in any one feed is 2 kg. If more than this is required feeds should be given in smaller amounts more frequently.

# GLYCAEMIC INDEX AND GLYCAEMIC RESPONSE

Carbohydrates do not all produce the same metabolic response once ingested by the horse. Many high starch feeds such as cereal straights and some mixes and cubes are absorbed and digested very quickly in the foregut giving a rapid rise in both blood sugar and insulin. Different feeds therefore have different effects on the horse's blood sugar levels. In addition spring pasture grass contains higher protein, sugars and/ or fructans and starch than later in the year and research has suggested these pastures can lead to marked fluctuations in blood glucose and insulin similar to those seen when cereal feeds are fed. The effects of these rapid rises and fluctuations in blood glucose and insulin in horses is thought to increase the risk of the development of growth related abnormalities such as DOD (developmental orthopaedic disease), insulin resistance and/or laminitis and obesity. Insulin sensitivity is also affected by the diet of horses. Insulin resistance is now thought to be an important predisposing factor for laminitis (see Chapter 12).

The concept of glycaemic index was developed over twenty-five years ago as a classification of foods based upon their ability to raise blood glucose in humans. These foods are now listed for humans. Foods with a high GI produce a higher and longer glucose peak in the blood following a meal of that food. Low GI foods release smaller amounts of glucose into the blood over a longer time. GI is a well known biological measurement applied to human foods.

This is now being tentatively applied to feeds for horses.

Until further information becomes available it would seem prudent to feed certain types of horses lower starch (<10% starch) and therefore lower GI feeds. The following should probably be fed low starch rations:

- Youngstock
- Obese horses and ponies
- Insulin resistant horses and ponies
- Laminitics or these prone to laminitis
- Veteran horses
- Horses prove to rhabdomyolysis.

Actual starch levels of feeds can be obtained from the feed manufacturer but coarse mixes (sweet feeds) are usually high in starch and therefore have a high GI, even many cool mixes are based upon large amounts of barley and are therefore high in starch.

Glycaemic response refers to the area under the graph when plasma glucose is plotted over time following a meal in humans. The glycaemic load refers to the GI of a food multiplied by the amount of available carbohydrate contained in the portion of food eaten. The glycaemic response of a coarse mix can be reduced by adding corn oil to the feed as this is thought to slow down digestion of starch.

Pelleted feeds have generally lower GI than coarse mixes although there are lower starch mixes now available.

## Oats (*Avena sativa*)

Oats are the traditional cereal of choice for horses and have been fed for centuries. Oats have a higher fibre content and lower starch than most other cereals making them safer to feed as they are less likely to be overfed and problems such as laminitis and colic are less likely (Figure 8.1 shows a cross section through an oat grain).

Also, oat starch is more digestible than many of the other cereal starches. This means that it is much more likely to be fully digested by enzymes in the small intestine and less likely to enter the hindgut undigested. If this happens, the starch may be rapidly fermented by hindgut microorganisms, often with serious consequences such as colic, diarrhoea or laminitis.

Oats are actually lower in energy than both maize and barley.

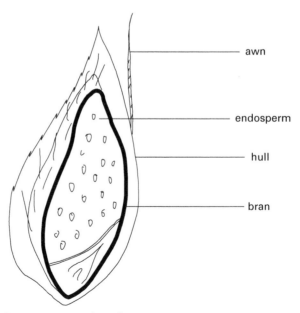

**Figure 8.1** Cross section through an oat grain.

## Naked oats (*Avena nuda* L)

This is a type of oat which readily loses its husk during threshing therefore there is no need for dehulling during the milling process. Naked oats are higher in crude protein and oil and are up to 30% higher in energy than conventional oats. Naked oats seem less likely to cause excitable behaviour sometimes associated with feeding oats, probably because of the higher oil content, providing energy in slow release form. However, the quantity fed should be restricted as the starch level will be higher (Table 8.1). When swapping to naked oats therefore less should be fed than with regular oats.

Oats may be fed whole to mature horses or those with good teeth (not youngstock). It is sometimes thought that oats are not digested very well as they can be seen in the droppings. In fact these are generally the outer indigestible husks and the middle part of the grain or endosperm has been digested.

Oats may be lightly processed mechanically such as rolling, bruising or crushing. Oats can vary tremendously in quality from plump starch filled grains to thin mainly fibre grains.

## Barley (*Hordeum vulgare*)

Barley is a smaller grain with a harder outer fibrous husk than oats, but it contains more energy and less fibre than oats. Because the outer covering is hard, barley needs to be processed in order to crack or break open the covering before it is fed to horses. Barley may be cooked, steamed, micronised or extruded; the purpose of all these processes is to make the starch more available and digestible to the horse.

**Table 8.1**  Nutrient compositions of commonly fed cereals.

|  | DE MJ/kg | CF % | CP % | Starch % | Oil% | Lysine % | Ca % | P % | Na % |
|---|---|---|---|---|---|---|---|---|---|
| Oats | 11.5 | 12.2 | 9.6 | 41.2 | 4.7 | 0.4 | 0.11 | 0.4 | 0.03 |
| Naked Oats | 14.5 | 4.5 | 14.0 | 60.0 | 10.0 | 0.6 | | | |
| Barley | 13.0 | 5.0 | 9.5 | 54.6 | 1.8 | 0.4 | 0.06 | 0.39 | 0.02 |
| Maize (corn) | 14.2 | 2.5 | 10.4 | 72.2 | 4.6 | 0.2 | 0.04 | 0.3 | 0.02 |

DE, digestible energy
CF, crude fibre
CP, crude protein

Boiling barley is traditional process in the winter months. Although this makes the starch more digestible, it will destroy any vitamins and, contrary to popular belief, will not warm the horse's core body temperature. Cold horses will benefit more from digestible fibre sources such as good quality forage as this produces heat within the gut as it is fermented.

There are several old wives' tales surrounding the feeding of barley, the most common myth being the assumption that barley puts fat on the horse's heart. Barley, if overfed, will put fat down all over the horse's body, it does not specifically target the heart.

## Maize (dent corn)

Dent corn or maize is mostly fed to livestock including horses (as opposed to popcorn or sweet corn). Maize is one of the most abundantly grown grains and the largest of the cereal grains.

Maize is higher in energy than any other cereal grain and it is also low in fibre. This means less should be fed as it is a potent energy source. It is therefore more likely to be overfed and cause digestive and behavioural problems. It tends to be more consistent in quality than oats. Maize needs to be processed before feeding, usually by cracking or micronising, as the starch is relatively difficult to digest in the small intestine and if larger quantities are fed it is more likely to result in hindgut acidosis problems.

## Wheat (*Triticum* spp)

Most wheat is used for human consumption, i.e. the bread making industry. This makes it an expensive raw material for the horse industry. It has approximately the same amount of energy as corn and is also low in fibre. Wheat also contains a substance called gluten, which gives dough its elasticity. Wheat may form a dough ball type mess in the horse's mouth particularly if ground wheat is fed. Wheat is most commonly fed to horses in the form of by-products such as bread meal or wheat bran.

## Wheat bran

Wheat bran consists of the outer husk of wheat after the flour has been removed. This is a fibrous type material containing some protein and a reverse calcium to phosphorus ratio.

Often simply called bran, wheat bran is another traditional feed for horses that has now become the subject of some dispute. Without doubt it must be fed with caution, since overfeeding or daily feeding significant amounts may result in metabolic health problems such as 'big head disease' or Miller's disease. The correct term is nutritional secondary hyperparathyroidism (NSHPT). This results from a reverse calcium to phosphorus ratio as bran contains high amounts of phosphorus. Wheat bran also contains phytate, which can considerably reduce the absorption of minerals in the digestive tract.

Bran is not a laxative for horses and should not be considered so. Although a small amount of wheat bran fed daily should not be harmful, there are other preferred fibre sources such as sugar beet pulp. In addition, a weekly bran mash is effectively a change of diet, which should be avoided at all costs. Wheat bran contains 16% protein and should not be fed at a rate of more than 0.5 kg per day per adult horse and this should be balanced for calcium with a calcium supplement such as limestone flour. Wheat bran is also expensive for the nutrients it provides and therefore sugar beet is a much better alternative.

All the cereals contain relatively low levels of calcium and sodium and high levels of phosphorus. These are important nutritional factors to correct. The protein quality is also relatively poor and in real terms cereals should be considered as simply a source of quick release energy. Cereals should therefore be fed with a balancer, a specific compound feed formulated to balance the nutrient deficiencies found in cereals. The balancer should be nutritionally formulated for either breeding stock or performance horses.

The energy from starch is a fast release energy source as starch is readily broken down to sugar in the small intestine where it is rapidly absorbed into the horse's bloodstream. The rise in blood sugar following a cereal 'meal' causes the insulin level to rise. These fluctuations in insulin are thought to have an effect on growth hormone in young stock. Insulin has a negative effect on maturing chondrocytes in the growth plates (see Chapter 6).

## PROCESSING CEREAL GRAINS

Whole grains are taken from the field and dried to a suitable moisture content before storage. Most grains, with the exception of oats as discussed previously, should be processed before feeding.

The purpose of mechanical processing is to break open the kernel so that once chewed and swallowed the digestive enzymes can access the starch and break it down in the small intestine before it gets to the hindgut where it may cause problems. Mechanical processing does not change the starch to make it more digestible. The cooking methods of processing break down the starch molecules – a process known as 'gelatinisation' – to make the starch more digestible.

Common physical processing methods include the following:

- Rolling – using rollers to smash the grain, this may be done with added steam
- Cracking – breaks the kernel into several pieces, more common with maize
- Crimping – slight flattening, such as carried out with oats
- Flaking – often heat treated with steam and then flattened.

Once cereals are broken open or cooked they start to deteriorate when exposed to air.

Micronising cereals consists of flaking and then heating in large machines similar to microwaves. The purpose of micronising is to break up the long starch chains so that the digestive enzymes can more easily break them down.

Extruding cereals involves cooking at high temperatures under great pressure, similar to popping corn (popcorn). Extrusion actually cooks the starch making it more digestible. Extruded feed may also be shaped through dyes and coloured and the end result may not look anything like the original cereal. Some horses have a problem with texture or mouth feel of extruded feeds and may reject them. Extruded cereals are very common in the dog food market!

## CEREAL/GRAIN BY-PRODUCTS

Many by-products are used in compound feeds and so it is appropriate to list them as they may be seen on labels in the list of ingredients:

- Oatfeed
- Wheatfeed
- Rice bran
- Molasses
- Beet pulp
- Soyabean hulls (soy hulls)
- Linseed meal
- Soyabean meal
- Sunflower seed meal
- Maize gluten feed
- Brewer's grains.

## Oatfeed

Oatfeed is a by-product of the commercial processing of oatmeal. It consists of oat hulls and hairs making it very high in fibre and so is often used in low energy, high fibre compound feeds. Oatfeed may also be added to coarse mixes as small pellets.

## Wheatfeed

Wheatfeed is a by-product of the wheat milling industry. It consists mainly of fragments of the outer skin of wheat and of particles of grain from which less of the starch containing endosperm has been removed than in bran. Wheatfeed is a general term applied to different grades of the outer fibrous coat and inner endosperm of wheat. The term 'middlings' was traditionally used and applied to the stage of the manufacturing process whereby it was extracted. Fine middlings applied to a by-product containing 25–60 g/kg crude fibre and more endosperm whereas coarse middlings applied to a product containing 60–85 g crude fibre and less endosperm. The endosperm contains more flour and therefore more starch and energy. Wheatfeed is commonly used in compound horse feeds.

## Rice bran

Although rice per se is not commonly fed to horses, rice bran is often added as a supplementary energy source. Rice bran consists of the outer covering of the rice grain with a small amount of hull. It may be white or brown and it is often used for horses as an energy source as it contains high levels of oil. Rice bran contains about the same fibre levels as oats but is much higher in oil at about 19–28%. Rice bran has reverse calcium to phosphorus ratio similar to all cereal grains and this should be taken into account when feeding. Rice bran contains a naturally occurring lipase, which is inactivated during processing to form stabilised rice bran, which is less likely to go rancid. Rice bran has a higher concentrate of phosphorus than wheat bran. Some commercial ricebran products have now added calcium to correct this imbalance. Therefore it is not recommended to be fed in large quantities.

Rice Bran contains gamma oryzanol an antioxidant with a supposed "steroidal" muscle building effect. This has not been supported by research as yet, and gamma oryzanol is a prohibited substance.

## Soyabean meal

Soyabean meal is often used in horse feeds as a good quality protein source owing to its high content of the essential amino acid lysine although it contains much lower levels of methionine. Soyabean meal or protein concentrate is obtained from heat treated, dehulled (husk removed by a process called decortication) soyabeans.

Whole soyabeans contain 15–20% oil. During processing, the soyabeans are toasted to remove various inhibitors such as trypsin, which inhibits the digestibility of protein; this is deactivated by heat treatment by toasting, roasting or extruding. The whole bean toasted product is known as toasted full fat soya. The protein content, by diluting with soyabean hulls is standardised at 44% or 50%.

Soyabean meal is also often solvent extracted and this is most widely used in horse feed manufacture in compound feeds and is also sometimes fed as a straight. It is high in energy and protein, very digestible and also palatable. Soyabean meal is therefore the most widely used vegetable protein concentrate.

Soya hulls, which consist of the outer husk of the soyabeans are often used as a fibre source as they contain low levels of lignin. These are often added to the low starch, high fibre and oil compound feeds as a good digestible fibre source.

## Sunflower seeds (*Helianthus annus*)

The thick black and white husk is generally removed by dehulling before further processing during the manufacturing process. Sunflower seeds are high in oil, protein and fibre, but extracted sunflower seed meal has had most of the oil removed and is a by-product of sunflower oil manufacture. Sunflower seed meal is not commonly fed as a straight but is included in some compound feeds.

## Linseed (*Linum usitassimum*)

Linseeds are also called flax seeds and so flax seed oil is actually linseed oil. Linseeds have been fed traditionally following prolonged boiling and simmering as a feed for helping coat condition and shine; linseed is now also being used as a good vegetable source of omega 3 fatty acids. Linseed oil is extracted from the linseed. The protein content is relatively low and it is deficient in the essential amino acid lysine.

Raw linseed may be a source of cyanide exposure. Linseeds are cyanogenic, but toxic effects are unknown from normal conditions of manufacture, which involve high temperature treatment. Although safer cultivars have been developed, unprocessed whole seeds and linseed cakes processed under low temperature can be toxic to horses. The potential cyanide yield can vary from 4 to 12 mmol/kg. Linseed contains the same cyanogenic glucosides as cassava.

If feeding linseed, the raw seeds should be soaked overnight and then boiled vigorously for a few minutes, then simmered until a jelly forms and left to cool before feeding. Linseed also contains mucilage (soluble fibre), which in the presence of water has the ability to swell, increasing its volume considerably. Mucilage is available to the hindgut bacteria even though horses do not have the enzymes to digest it. This bulking ability can be extremely beneficial to the digestive tract of horses with chronic digestive problems.

## Molasses

Molasses is a syrupy residue that is a major by-product of the sugar manufacturing process; most molasses comes from sugar cane: 100 kg of refined sugar results in the production of between 25 and 50 kg molasses. Molasses is also produced from the extraction of sugar from sugar beet and it may also be derived from other crops such as sorghum and corn.

Molasses is essentially an energy source and is a widely used feedstuff for horses as it is sweet tasting. It can also be used to reduce dust in compound feeds and as a binder for pellets and cubes. It may be fed separately to help mask medicines and supplements in the feed. The total sugars in cane molasses and beet molasses are:

• Cane molasses – 48–54% total sugars
• Beet molasses – 48–52% total sugars.

Molasses is typically added to compound feeds and chaff products often at an inclusion rate of less than 10%. Molasses is also a good source of potassium.

## Sugar beet pulp

This is the residue left after extraction of sugar from sugar beet. Molasses is often added before drying of the end product, which may then be sold as shred or pellets. If molasses has been added the end product will be called molassed sugar beet; if not it will be called unmolassed, which is often preferred for horses. Sugar beet pellets and shreds should be soaked before feeding even though this is not often recommended in the USA for shreds. There is also a micronised beet pulp product, which requires a very short soak time, i.e. roughly ten minutes, which is very popular.

Recommended soaking times are given below:

- Sugar beet shreds – 12 hours' soaking
- Sugar beet pellets – 24 hours' soaking
- Micronised beet pulp flakes –10 minutes' soaking.

Sugar beet is very palatable and is often used to mask the taste of supplements in the feed. It can also be fed warm to make an appetising mash in the cold months and given to mares that have just foaled. Sugar beet shreds are often included in compound feeds as a good fibre source but these do not need soaking.

Sugar beet is a very useful feed for horses, as it is rich in calcium and low in phosphorus. It contains high levels of highly digestible fibre sources including pectins and so is an excellent medium energy feed for horses. In fact, up to 4.5 kg (dry weight) of beet pulp could be fed per day but this is not common. It should be supplemented with a balanced vitamin and mineral, and essential amino acids supplement such as a good forage balancer. It should not be fed as the sole feed.

## Brewer's grains

This is a by-product of the brewing industry obtained usually from the drying of residues of barley malt and/or other malted and unmalted cereals and other starchy products.

## Maize gluten feed

This is a by-product of the wet manufacture of maize starch and glucose. This is made up of gluten and bran and the oil-extracted germ. Maize screenings and other starch-derived products may also be added at a rate of no more than 15%. Maize gluten feed is high in energy and protein and is often added to compound feeds for horses.

## Peas and beans

These are protein rich seeds of legumes and are good sources of the essential amino acid lysine. They must be heat treated before feeding to horses. Steam flaked peas are often added to coarse mixes to add colour. Beans and peas contain higher levels of protein and also starch and so should only be fed in limited quantities.

## Vegetable oil

This is simply oil extracted from plants, e.g. corn oil from corn, sunflower oil from sunflower seeds, linseed oil from linseed or flax seed, and rice bran oil from rice bran.

# COMPOUND FEEDS

Compound feeds are manufactured feeds usually in the form of cubes/pellets or coarse mixes. Compound feeds have been fed to horses for many years now. They can be divided roughly into four groups:

- Complete cubes or coarse mixes
- Concentrate cubes or coarse mixes
- Balancers – pellets or coarse mixes, or protein concentrates
- Chaff (alfalfa/hay/straw) or fibre based mixes with added ingredients and premix.

Complete cubes or coarse mixes are fed alone without forage and are designed to replace both the hay and concentrates in the ration. High fibre and low energy, they tend to be used for overweight ponies or when hay is scarce. Care must be taken with complete cubes, as the fibre length is often too short for horses. Horses need a minimum length of fibre for efficient gut function. Some horses on high fibre cubes may chew wood in their search for long fibre. Such cubes should therefore be fed with a good quality chaff.

## Concentrate cubes or coarse mixes/sweet feeds

These provide a balanced diet for all types of horses and are designed to be fed with forage and water. Different formulations are made for horses with different needs. High protein feeds for growing stock, high energy feeds for working horses and low energy feeds for resting horses or those in light work. There are many different types now available to suit every need, even for veterans. Compound feeds are also available for horses prone to tying up and laminitis for example.

The deficiencies of straights are balanced by the addition of a premix to provide a nutritionally balanced feed. Cool cubes or mixes may be oat free but may still contain barley, for example, and be high in starch. Low starch cool feeds are preferred.

## Advantages of compound feeds

- Convenient
- Scientifically formulated to provide balanced nutrients
- Quality control
- Improved shelf life
- Mycotoxin binders often added
- Dustfree
- Palatable
- Easy storage
- No waste.

Coarse mixes or sweet feeds look appetising like muesli, however some horses are able to filter out individual ingredients and tend to leave the important premix pellets for example. For appearance, coarse mixes or sweet feeds contain high levels of cereal straights including flaked maize and peas, which can make them high in starch. Many coarse mixes also contain chaff such as alfalfa, herbs and dried carrots/apples. Low starch coarse mixes contain lower cereal amounts and tend to look less appetising to the 'feeder' but are better for the horse. Cubes however tend to be lower in starch.

Compound feeds are nutritionally formulated to be fed at a set rate per day and also assume adequate forage intake. Therefore if feeding at less than the recommended amount, vitamin and mineral intake and quality amino acids may be too low and a balancer is preferred (see below).

Cubes or pellets are made by first grinding down the ingredients then binding them together and pushing the ground material under pressure through a dye to form the pellet. They are cheaper to make than coarse mixes and tend to be more consistent. They should be fed with a handful of chaff to ensure the horse chews them thoroughly.

All compound feeds must by law, declare certain ingredients, and these are a very useful reference for comparison of different products.

Quality compound feeds are expensive compared with straights, owing to the high costs of good raw materials, nutritionists, higher quality protein, higher specification premixes and analytical equipment, not to mention the plant machinery and quality control.

## Balancer cubes/balancer coarse mixes

These are higher in protein and designed to balance a straight such as oats or to balance mineral deficiencies in forage. They are actually

**Table 8.2** Comparison of a typical balancer with a standard compound feed.

| | Working mix (12% crude protein 10 MJ/kg DE) | | Balancer (24% Crude Protein 11 MJ/kg DE) |
|---|---|---|---|
| **500 g** | **Daily Intake**<br>60 g protein<br>5 MJ/kg DE<br>(**not** providing adequate vitamins and minerals at this intake) | **500 g** | **Daily Intake**<br>120 g protein<br>5.5 MJ/kg DE<br>(should provide balanced vitamins and minerals at this intake) |
| **3 kg** | **Daily Intake**<br>360 g protein<br>30 MJ/kg DE<br>(should provide balanced vitamins and minerals at this intake) | **3 kg** | N/A should not be fed at higher than recommended amount |

**Table 8.3** Nutrient content of some typical compound feeds.

| | CP% | Oil % | MAD Fibre % | Ca g/kg | P g/kg | Lysine g/kg | DE MJ/kg |
|---|---|---|---|---|---|---|---|
| Horse& pony nuts | 9–11 | 2.5 | 16 | 0.7 | 0.35 | 0.4 | 10 |
| Performance mix/ cubes | 12 | 3.5 | 5 | 0.9 | 0.45 | 0.75 | 13.5 |
| Stud diet | 15 | 3 | 8.5 | 1.2 | 0.65 | 0.75 | 13.5 |
| Racing mix/cubes | 13 | 8.5 | 8 | 0.9 | 0.5 | 0.6 | 14 |

'concentrated' compound feeds. An example is a 50:50 oats to oat balancer mix. Half the concentrate ration is oats, which is nutritionally unbalanced, and the other half oat balancer, to balance the deficiencies in the oats. The combination results in a balanced ration when fed with forage. Forage balancers are now very common as they tend to be lower in energy and are therefore extremely useful for overweight horses and ponies and those that maintain weight on forage alone. Fed in much smaller quantities, typically 500 g (or about 1 lb) per day and no more, these feeds are more like a supplement than a typical concentrate feed. Because they are more concentrated nutritionally than the normal compound feeds, protein and energy levels are higher, however smaller amounts are fed (Table 8.2). It is important not to overfeed balancers and follow the feeding guideline.

## CHOOSING A FEED

Compound feeds are specifically formulated for certain classes and types of horses in various stages of work or stage of the breeding cycle, etc. Nutritionists take the raw materials available and balance any

**Table 8.4**   Comparison of four typical horse and pony cube products (2008).

|  | A | B | C | D |
|---|---|---|---|---|
| (Energy) DE MJ/kg | 10 | 8.5 | 10 | 10 |
| (Protein) CP% | 10 | 10 | 11.5 | 10 |
| Fibre % | 15 | 16 | 11 | 17 |
| Vit A IU/kg | 10,000 | 10,000 | 10,000 | 8000 |
| Vit D IU/kg | 1500 | 1500 | 2000 | 1000 |
| Vit E IU/kg | 100 | 80 | 50 | 75 |

deficiencies to match nutrient requirements for each feed, providing a nutritionally balanced product usually formulated to complement average quality hay//haylage/pasture. Different balancers, for example, are formulated to complement forage or cereals. Not all compound feeds are the same, however, and quality control and ingredients'/nutrient content can differ widely among a group of products designed for the same purpose, e.g. horse and pony cubes. Table 8.4 shows a range of horse and pony feeds and compares basic nutrient levels to give an indication.

It is a good idea to compare feed labels and prices and also the reputations of feed manufacturers when making a choice. Larger feed compounders, for example, are able to purchase higher quality raw materials and in fact can even instruct farmers as to their precise needs when growing the crops in the field. This provides consistency and superior quality control of ingredients which is vital.

Feed labels are a useful tool and give a good indication, for example the vitamin content can be compared between different horse and pony feeds. Higher vitamin content sometimes means the cost is slightly higher, but the product may be better quality.

Feeding straights and balancing them with a compounded balancer feed is quite common and allows traditional straight cereals to be fed, although it is important to feed the recommended amount of balancer to maintain a balanced nutrient intake.

## Compound feeds

Horse and pony feeds and 'cool' non-heating feeds are formulated to be fed to horses at maintenance and doing light work. These can contain highly variable amounts of starch depending upon the cereal content which varies from 7% to 25%. The feed company should be contacted to ascertain the starch content prior to making a choice as high starch feeds could actually cause and exacerbate over-excitable behaviour even though the product is labelled as a cool feed.

The choice of product will depend upon the individual horse and its requirements but the following are available usually as both cubes and coarse mixes or sweet feeds

- Horse and pony – cool cubes/mixes, quiet cubes/mixes herbal, leisure feeds – high fibre, low energy for horses in light work or resting
- Chaff based compound feeds – low /medium energy
- Conditioning – high oil/fibre, high energy for horses needing condition
- Performance – endurance, polo, show jumping, eventing, dressage, medium to high energy
- Racing – balancers, cubes, mixes, high energy for increased nutrient needs
- Stud – foal creep, stud cubes/mixes, stallion, high energy
- Yearling – breaking and prepping, low starch, low-medium energy
- Balancers – stud, forage and cereal, low energy
- Veteran – medium energy, medium fibre
- Health specific problems – laminitis, tying up (ERS), convalescents etc.

It is important to make the right choice matching the needs of horses to the correct feed.

## Feed/mineral blocks

Feed blocks or keep blocks are most commonly made from cereals, vegetable proteins, and minerals and vitamins and sometimes herbs bound together by molasses, often left in a plastic container to be placed in the field. They tend to contain low levels of nutrients such as protein, energy and vitamins and minerals. Theoretically these products are formulated to be placed in the field for horses and ponies to self consume, providing additional nutrients particularly in the winter. However, they are also commonly given to stabled horses and horses on poor or limited pasture and this can lead to severe problems due to over-consumption from boredom and/or hunger. Molasses has a very sweet taste and this can also promote over-consumption. It is vital that the recommended daily dose is not exceeded. If the block is not molasses based horses are far less likely to over-consume but consumption must still be monitored.

For example, the recommended dose for a feed block is 150 g per day for a 15 kg block (15,000 g) this should theoretically last:

- 1 horse = 15,000 g/150 = 100 days
- 2 Horses = 15,000 g/300 = 50 days
- 4 Horses = 15,000 g/600 = 25 days.

If four horses consume the block in 17 days, say, then another block should not be given until 25 days after the original block was put in the field. This is very important if toxicity problems are to be avoided. If one horse is seen to over- consume the block should be removed permanently. In practice, often one horse may over-consume and the others under-consume, making it very difficult indeed to monitor individual intake. These blocks should not be given with compound feeds when the compound feed is fed at the recommended level.

Monensin is an antibiotic used extensively in the beef and dairy industries to improve growth rates, where it is marketed under the name Rumensin. Monensin is extremely toxic and can be fatal when fed to horses. It is important therefore not to give feed or mineral blocks (or any other feed for that matter) formulated and manufactured for cattle to horses.

## Mineral blocks

Mineral blocks are generally salt based and contain additional minerals particularly trace minerals. These can be useful for horses at pasture including breeding stock and, as they are salt based, they are less likely to be over-consumed. None the less, intake should be monitored particularly if breeding stock also have access to creep feeds or are fed high levels of concentrates. A pure salt block is preferred in these circumstances. High copper blocks are also unnecessary when stud rations are being fed.

## SHELF LIFE OF FEEDS

Many feedstuffs will begin to deteriorate as soon as the sealed bag is opened and the feed is exposed to oxygen. Cereals should be kept in a dry environment once opened, to prolong their shelf life. Whole, unprocessed cereals may be stored for up to 12 months. Processed grains are drier and have a shelf life of about six months, until the bag is opened. Once opened, the contents should be used within two weeks.

Unopened feeds will eventually become stale and disintegrate. The Feedingstuffs Regulations permit the addition of limited amounts of synthetic antioxidants such as ethoxyquine, BHA *butylated hydroxyanisole* and BHT *butylated hydroxytoluene*. These substances are safe to add and are able to extend the shelf life of the feed. For feed manufacturers this can be very helpful as feed is often transported around the world. For whole unadulterated cereals, however, they can remain quite stable for much longer periods of time, particularly if stored in appropriate conditions at moisture levels of less than 13.5%. It is the mechanical processing which begins the process of deterioration.

Feeds should not be fed after the use-by date. Vitamins naturally present or those that have been added via a premix may have lost their activity. Out of date feed can also be unpalatable for horses. Feed that has any evidence of mould should be discarded and should never be fed to horses.

## MYCOTOXINS

The word mycotoxin stems from the Greek word 'mykes' meaning mould and 'toxicum' meaning poison. Mycotoxins are toxic secondary metabolites produced by fungi growing on crops in the field, during handling and in storage. Mycotoxins are capable of causing disease that may be potentially fatal. Fungi only produce mycotoxins under favourable conditions such as specific moisture levels, oxygen levels in the air and temperature, in other words the presence of fungi does not necessarily indicate the presence of mycotoxins. There are thousands of different species of fungi, but only a relatively small number (about 100 species) have the ability to produce mycotoxins.

Mycotoxins are often found in cereals such as oats, barley, maize and wheat and their by-products. They may also be found on pasture and in conserved forage in certain environmental conditions. Mycotoxins enter the horse via feed, forage or bedding. In fact mycotoxins are odourless and horses cannot taste them in feed, making ingestion more likely. Ingestion of contaminated feed or forage and inhalation from mould-infested bedding are all-important causes of exposure. Low-level intakes of mycotoxins over long periods are likely to produce chronic toxicological symptoms. This may affect athletic performance and breeding capability possibly without actual obvious disease symptoms. General symptoms such as loss of appetite, weight loss, unthriftiness, poor performance, increased susceptibility to infectious diseases, reduced growth rates and poor breeding performance, for example increased red bag delivery, may all be associated with chronic myco-toxin intake. Because mycotoxins negatively affect equine performance and health, mycotoxin control is crucial for equine welfare and feed safety reasons.

Historically, human cases of ergotism or St Anthony's fire have been described in Europe since the Middle Ages and are now known to be caused by mycotoxins produced in rye by the mould *Claviceps purpurea*. Since then many more mycotoxins, such as trichothecenes, zearale-none, ochratoxins and fumonisins have been discovered.

The term mycoses refers to actual growth of fungi on the animal host whereas the term mycotoxicoses refers to disease caused by ingestion or inhalation of toxic fungal metabolites by the animal.

Fungi may be found on pasture or in cereal grains in varying amounts each year depending upon the environmental conditions. A cooler wetter season is more likely to result in greater fungal contamina-tion of crops. High moisture levels will increase fungal growth and cooler temperatures will result in the formation of mycotoxins by the fungi.

Mycotoxins vary greatly in their severity. As horses are hindgut fermentors it is thought they may be more susceptible to the effects of mycotoxins than ruminants, which are able to degrade many mycotox-ins in the rumen. Horses (unlike ruminants) will take mycotoxins into the body following ingestion of contaminated feed or forage. Eventually the mycotoxins will enter the small intestine where they may exert their effects on the intestinal wall or be absorbed into the horse's body via the blood.

Mycotoxins have been implicated in causing colic, organ disease (liver, kidneys) reduced growth rate, respiratory problems, poor feed efficiency, reduced fertility and even death. General symptoms (reduced performance, impaired immunity) are seen when dealing with moderate mycotoxin levels, while symptoms caused by higher mycotoxin levels are often more specific and obvious. Further comp-lications in mycotoxicosis diagnoses can be caused by secondary symptoms resulting from opportunistic disease related to the suppres-sion of the immune system following mycotoxin exposure. In addi-tion, mycotoxicoses increase the horse's vulnerability to microbial diseases.

Mycotoxins thought to cause problems in equine health are:

- Aflatoxin
- T2 toxin
- DON

- Zearalenone
- Fumonisins
- Ergovaline.

## Mycotoxin binders

As the risk of mycotoxicosis is very difficult to predict or evaluate, prevention strategies should be put in place. These should aim at minimising mycotoxin formation in the field and during storage.

Cleanliness is vital and all feed bins and utensils should be cleaned regularly and kept dry. Mouldy or out of date feeds should not be fed even though they may not necessarily contain mycotoxins. Hay and chaff products must be properly harvested and dried. Feed should preferably be kept within the bag until just before use and once opened stored in a cool dry place free from extreme temperature fluctuations. Bedding in stables should be cleaned out thoroughly and deep litter bedding is more likely to contain fungi. Thorough cleaning of areas around the mangers is also important.

Most feed manufacturers regularly test the raw materials and finished feed and many now add mycotoxin binders to the feeds to help insure against possible mycotoxin presence. Speciality feed additives, known as mycotoxin adsorbents or binding agents, are the most common approach to prevent and treat mycotoxicosis in horses. It is believed that the agents bind to the mycotoxin preventing them from being absorbed. The mycotoxins and the binding agent are excreted in the manure.

Mycotoxin adsorbents offer an attractive short-term solution to the challenge of mycotoxin-contaminated horse feeds.

## FEED LABELLING REQUIREMENTS

There are a vast number of feeds and supplements available for horses today and horse owners need to be able to distinguish between them when making the right choices to suit the needs of their horses. Feed manufacturers must legally supply certain information to the consumer on the labels or feedbags and supplements. This includes chaff products. These legal requirements are the same as those stipulated for farm animals being produced for food. Under domestic legislation, only horses that are farmed for meat, or for their hides, or used to farm agricultural land can be said to be agricultural animals. This follows from the Agricultural Act 1947, however EU legislation treats the horse as a food producing animal. This reflects the fact that horse meat is eaten in certain EU Member States. Some manufacturers of horse feed and supplements may also supply additional details that are not legal requirements and are simply aimed at helping horse owners make a more informed choice. The laws and information required vary between countries and here we refer to those used in the UK. The information required is given in the Feeding Stuffs Regulations 2005 and this is a very lengthy document.

## Statutory statement

The statutory statement must be printed on the bag by law and must be clearly readable in English and separate from the rest of the information supplied by the manufacturer (Figure 8.2). It includes:

1. Name of the feed – product name and brand - what type of horse the feed is intended for
2. Description of the feed or purpose statement and the species of animal for which it has been made – i.e. 'complete feeding stuff'

### 0625323 GAIN STUD CUBES

PROTEIN 15.0%. OIL 4.5%. FIBRE 10.0%. ASH 7.50%. MOISTURE 14.00%.
VITAMIN A 15000IU/KG VITAMIN D3 2000IU/KG
ALPHA-TOCOPHEROL (VIT E) 250IU/KG
COPPER (AS CU SULPHATE PEN.) 10.00mg/kg
COPPER (AS CU CHELATE OF AMINO ACIDS) 15.00mg/kg
SELENIUM (AS NA SELENITE) 0.30mg/kg
Ingredients used in descending order by weight are:-
WHEATFEED, OATS, SOYA (bean) HULLS[2], SUNFLOWERSEED EXTRACTED,
BARLEY, CANE MOLASSES, LUCERNE, SOYA (bean), Extracted,Toasted [2], MAIZE,
CALCIUM CARBONATE, PALM OIL, SOYA (bean) OIL[2], SODIUM CHLORIDE, BINDER,
MINERALS, MONO-DICALCIUM PHOSPHATE, MYCOCURB, YEAST.

AT TIME OF MANUFACTURE THE FOLLOWING WAS/WERE ADDED:-
Saccharomyces cerevisiae CBS 493.94  giving 2*1000000000 CFU/kg.feed.
[2] Produced from genetically modified Soya Beans.

**COMPLEMENTARY FEEDINGSTUFF**
Feed to all breeding horses along with forage and water.
Feed in regular small meals (max 0.5kg/meal/100kg bodyweight).
Provide adequate forage (min 1.0kg/day /100kg bodyweight).
Adjust feeding rates for body weight, body condition, forage quality and workload.
Feed as instructed on the bag and label. Do not feed to livestock other than indicated.
Store in a cool dry place. Use before the "Best before date" on the bag or label.

| FEEDING GUIDELINES (Thoroughbreds ) | | | |
|---|---|---|---|
| | Pregnant mares | Lactating mares | Barren mares |
| Stud Cubes (kg/head/day) | 2.0-4.0 | 4.5-6.5 | 1.5 |

BEST BEFORE 14.Apr.2009
Manufactured 120 days before the minimum storage life expiry date indicated.
Manufactured for Glanbia Foods Society Ltd., Glanbia House, Kilkenny.
Approval No.:  aIEWX100145.
Version 43      UFAS No. 1034 - renewal date 28/06/2009
~~~~~~~~~~~~~~~~~~~~ Information Only ~~~~~~~~~~~~~~~~~~~~
Protected Copper added @ 15 mg/kg.

**Figure 8.2** Statuatory feed label. Courtesy of Gain Horse Feeds.

therefore no other feed required or 'complementary compound feeding stuff' to be fed in addition to forage (pasture and/or hay/haylage) to horses

3. Name and address of registered office
4. Ingredients in descending order, i.e. from highest amount to lowest. These may be listed in generic terms such as grain products or by-products, plant protein products, animal protein products, forage products, etc., or as specific listings such as oats, barley, soyabean meal, etc.
5. Best before or 'use-by' date
6. Directions for use
7. Net weight – this varies mostly between15 kg and 25 kg.
8. Batch number – this should be kept if there is a problem to report to the feed manufacturer
9. Registration number of manufacturer
10. Nutrient analysis – manufacturers currently have to legally declare the following: crude protein, oil, fibre, ash, calcium if greater then 5%, phosphorus if greater than 2%. Moisture if greater than 14%.
11. Additives – amount and what form added
    • Vitamins A, D and E – those naturally in the feed ingredients and those added. Vitamins A and D should include the name of the vitamin and active substance level. Vitamin E should include the alpha tocopherol level Preservatives, colours, antioxidants
    • Copper – naturally present in the feed ingredients and any added
    • Enzymes if present
    • Microorganisms – such as probiotics, identification and file number of each strain and the number given in CFU/kg (colony forming units), EC registration number, projected shelf life of microorganisms.

## Prohibited substances

Under the Horseracing Regulatory Authority's rules and those of the International Equestrian Federation (FEI), BSJA and British Equestrian Federation (BEF) it is strictly forbidden to give any stimulant, sedative or substance other than a normal nutrient to a competing horse. Detection of such a substance in the blood, sweat, saliva or urine of the horse, will lead to immediate disqualification. Obviously these prohibited substances are not deliberately included in feeds, but accidental contamination can and does occur particularly as the detectable levels required to invoke disqualification are so minute (parts per million or parts per billion). The list of substances is long and covers those that affect all the systems of the horse either by stimulation or other means and includes painkillers, which allow horses to compete. The BEF rules also apply to the use of herbs for calming or stimulating and are looking into possible testing for herbal substances in the near future.

The substances that are mostly tested for in feeds are theobromine, caffeine and its metabolite theophylline. Feedstuffs can be inadvertently contaminated when carried in bulk containers that have previously carried cargos such as coffee, cocoa and tea.

If feeding competition horses, concentrate feed should be chosen that has been routinely tested for the presence of prohibited substances and compound feeds and supplements are labelled as such. If feeding straights this should be checked with the supplier, although unless they have been purchased through a reputable compounder it is unlikely they have been tested. Keep the feedbags so that batch numbers are available if there is a problem. Chaff products are less likely to be tested, as forage products are much less likely to be contaminated.

## NUTRIENT ANALYSIS OF FEEDSTUFFS

The system of analysis most commonly used historically is called the proximate analysis of food devised roughly one hundred years ago, which divides the food sample into six fractions namely:

- Moisture
- Ash – mainly essential elements, minerals
- Crude protein – proteins, amino acids, B vitamins, amines, nitrates, etc.
- Ether extract – fats, oils, vitamins A,D,E and K
- Crude fibre – cellulose, hemicelluloses, lignin
- Nitrogen free extractives – cellulose, hemicelluloses, lignin, sugars, fructans, starch, pectins, organic acids, water soluble vitamins, etc.

The following may be seen on feed labels, i.e. ash, oil, crude fibre and crude protein, but they are not ingredients, they are simply analytical figures as assessed in laboratories of the finished feed.

More recently nutritionists have argued that some of these tests are out of date and so other analytical procedures are now determined in addition to or instead of nitrogen free extract and crude fibre. However the above details are still used on the statutory statement.

The NDF or Neutral Detergent Fibre includes cellulose, hemicellulose and lignin and is considered a measure of the plant cell wall material. ADF or Acid Detergent Fibre level includes lignin, cellulose and silica. There is a good correlation between ADF and digestibility, also the higher the ADF the lower the energy. In the UK this procedure has been changed slightly to give MADF or modified Acid Detergent Fibre. More importantly new technology such as IR (infrared) spectrophotometry has enabled laboratories to more accurately provide information without time consuming physical tests.

Other tests available include:

- Fatty acid analysis
- Amino acid analysis
- GMO testing
- Microbiology testing
- Mycotoxins Analysis
- Tests for sugar and starch
- Minerals
- Vitamins.

---

**Summary points**

- An understanding of the most common feedstuffs and the nutrients they supply to horses is vital.
- A feedstuff may be defined as any component of the horse's diet that serves some useful function.
- Concentrates are fed to increase energy supply or energy density.
- Different feeds have different effects on the horse's blood sugar levels.
- Most grains should be processed before feeding with the exception of oats.
- Feed labels allow comparisons to be made between different horse and pony feeds.
- Feeds should not be fed after the use-by date.
- Mycotoxins present a health threat to horses and are often found in cereals such as oats, barley, maize and wheat and their by-products and pasture.
- Mycotoxin adsorbents offer an attractive short-term solution to the challenge of mycotoxin-contaminated horse feeds.

# Feed Supplements, Additives and Nutraceuticals

A large number of supplements and additives are available for horses. These are supplied in many forms such as powders, granules liquids, syrups and oils. Additives are commonly added to feeds and are described as non-nutritive ingredients that stimulate growth or production, improve feed efficiency or utilisation or benefit the health or metabolism of the horse. Additives include antioxidants and preservatives, enzymes, flavours, pellet binders and anticaking agents.

Supplements include a huge range of products such as:

- Broad spectrum – e.g. multivitamin and mineral supplements
- Oils – e.g. linseed, soya, cod liver oil, omega 3 supplements
- Vitamins – e.g. E, C, B group vitamins, biotin
- Iron (haematinics) – B complex, copper
- Copper
- Calcium, e.g. limestone flour
- Sodium zeolite
- Epsom salts
- Prebiotics
- Probiotics
- Yeasts
- Performance enhancing products.

Feed supplements and nutraceuticals often target specific problem areas such as:

- Hooves – biotin, methionine, zinc, calcium
- Mobility and joints – glucosamine, chondroitin, omega 3's, MSM, hyaluronic acid (HA), glutamine, cider vinegar, cod liver oil, green lipped muscle extract
- Respiratory – vitamin C, antioxidants, herbs
- Calming – B complex, L-tryptophan, magnesium, herbs
- Digestion – prebiotics, yeast, buffers

- Skin, coat and condition– omega 3 fatty acids, zinc
- Haematinics – iron, B complex, copper
- Immune function – antioxidants, echinacea, yeast, prebiotics
- Performance – creatine, DMG, L-carnitine.

Nutraceutical is a broad term that encompasses any supplement or additive fed for perceived health benefit as opposed to nutrients. Nutraceuticals are not nutrients even though the term is derived from 'nutrient' + 'pharmaceutical'. Examples of nutraceuticals include anti-oxidants, antacids, probiotics and preprobiotics, joint and digestive supplements, enzymes, performance enhancing products such as DMG (dimethylglycine) and creatine, yeast culture and herbs. Often they are sold as complementary feeding stuffs but it must be stressed that they are not nutrients. If EU laws are enforced in the UK products will require licensing and, owing to the high cost of this process, some may disappear from the market place. This does not include pharmaceutical drugs that are fully licensed, researched and prescribed by vets. There is plenty of anecdotal evidence to support nutraceuticals but this will not be enough if new EU legislation is applied.

In addition to the active ingredients, supplements often contain other substances such as fillers, binders and extenders. Fillers increase the volume of material for easier measuring and dosing.

## WHEN MIGHT SUPPLEMENTS BE REQUIRED?

Some supplements are given on a short-term basis, often by vets or nutritionists to help with known short-term problems. Examples of this would be where horses are post-viral and may include B vitamin sup-plements or tonics, and herbs such as echinacea.

Before adding a supplement or additive the feeding programme should be properly evaluated to see whether or not there is an actual need. Forage analysis is important so that any deficiencies found can be made good in the concentrate part of the diet or given as a supple-ment. Some forage samples may show high levels of certain minerals such as iron and/or manganese. If, for example, an iron supplement is also being fed in addition to maximal amounts of compound feed then copper availability could be greatly reduced.

There is plenty of ongoing research concerning vitamins and their importance with varying results particularly when looking at immune function.

Certainly there are times when working horses and breeding stock are stressed or fatigued and the immune system becomes compromised. These horses may benefit from supplementation. Vitamin C is made by the horse's liver but at times of stress or illness it may be insufficient and horses may be fed 10 g per day for a short time. Horses with healthy hindgut microbes are able to make their own B vitamins and these are absorbed to an unknown extent by the horse. However, ill or stressed horses and those following antibiotic therapy may benefit from B complex supplementation and prebiotics.

These should help to re-establish a healthy microbial balance. Horses with loose droppings may also benefit from B complex vitamins.

Great care should be taken when adding supplements particularly relating to dosage rates and total ration content (including concentrates and forage) as overfeeding of fat-soluble vitamins and also some minerals may lead to toxicity problems. Harmful effects through over-supplementation or nutrient interactions are common and advice should be sought from the nutritionist or vet. Most compound feeds for working horses and breeding stock are already formulated to meet nutrient requirements when fed at recommended levels and so supplementation is likely to be unnecessary and expensive.

## HERBS

There is an abundance of herbal preparations on the market today. These are available for every type of condition or ailment ranging from depression to inflammation and digestive aids to perceived 'PMT' in moody mares. A number of herbs may also contain alkaloids and are therefore of questionable safety. Feeding herbs in order to prevent or treat disease defines the herb as a drug requiring legal regulation. There is a lack of scientific data and research generally regarding the use of herbs in horses. Toxicity, whether acute or chronic, may be a problem when herbal preparations are fed over the long term and extrapolation of data from humans or animals is not reliable.

Herbs tend to be slow growing and deep rooted and include a wide range of natural plants thought to have therapeutic properties.

Some herbs already have safety questions, for example comfrey, which has been shown to cause liver damage in humans and animals and as such is no longer used in human or equine supplements. Herbal extracts are prepared by concentrating the active part of the herb; these seem to be more widely available in human medicine. Because they are often standardised the quality will usually be superior. As many herbs contain quite potent chemicals care should be taken when feeding to pregnant mares and youngstock. Always follow the feeding recommendations given on the label. Some information on commonly used herbs is given below.

## Aloe vera (*Aloe vera barbadensis*)

This is a succulent plant from Africa. There are about 200 different species but only about four of these are used for their medicinal properties of which the most useful is *Aloe vera barbadensis*. The gel is commonly used topically for sunburn, insect bites and minor wounds as it is purported to have anti-inflammatory, antiseptic, antibacterial and antifungal properties.

Aloe vera may also be used as a digestive supplement but should not be fed to pregnant mares as it is thought it may stimulate uterine contractions increasing risk of foetal loss.

## Devil's claw (*Harpagophytum procumbens*)

This is a desert plant from South Africa, the tubers of which contain active compounds such as harpagoside. Devil's claw is thought to have natural anti-inflammatory properties, helping to reduce pain from arthritis, muscle pain or sports injuries.

## Echinacea (*Echinacea purpurea* – Purple coneflower)

Echinacea is thought to stimulate the immune system by increasing the number of white blood cells. Echinacea is also thought to help prevent and treat upper respiratory tract infections. It contains flavonoids that have antioxidant properties. Echinacea contains several unique substances known as echinacins. This herb is used to boost the immune system and help to ward off common viruses such as the cold in humans. A study showed some effects of feeding echinacea to horses. Echinacea was shown to have several effects:

- Increase in circulating or white blood cells
- Significant increase in the size and number of circulating erythrocytes or red blood cells
- Increase in haemoglobin.

These trials were able to scientifically support the immune stimulating effect and haematinic effects of feeding echinacea to horses. However, these trials were carried out on mature horses, not youngstock or pregnant mares. Echinacea should not be fed to pregnant mares until proper research endorses its use during pregnancy.

## Garlic (*Allium sativum*)

Garlic has been used for many years and is known for its antibacterial, antiseptic, antiviral and antioxidant properties.

The main active substance in garlic is allicin which gives the garlic clove its characteristic strong smell. Allicin is found in whole garlic cloves as an odourless precursor known as alliin. Once garlic is crushed or sliced, an enzyme called alliinase breaks down alliin into the strong smelling allicin.

Allicin has a half-life in the blood of less than one minute, it is highly unstable. Researchers therefore looked for another compound within garlic that may have antibacterial properties while being more stable. A garlic metabolite known as allyl mercaptan was found to be more stable.

Garlic is considered a natural and 'safe' herb. However, horses that consumed freeze-dried garlic at a rate of more than 0.2 mg/kg body-weight in two meals per day, showed signs of oxidative damage to red blood cells. (This equates to 100 mg in each of two meals for a 500 kg horse.) After removal of the garlic supplement the horses' blood parameters improved after 4–5 weeks. In addition, horses voluntarily ate toxic doses of freeze-dried garlic for 71 days at a rate of 0.25 g/kg bodyweight twice per day. This equates to 125 g freeze-dried garlic twice per day or 250 g per day.

## Milk thistle (*Silybum marianum*)

The seeds of milk thistle contain a unique and powerful mixture of antioxidants called silymarin. Silymarin is thought to help protect liver cells and therefore may be useful for horses suffering from ragwort poisoning or liver damage. Silymarin may increase levels of an important liver enzyme, glutathione.

## Valerian (*Valerian officinalis*)

This herb is thought to have calming properties, its roots contain unique compounds such as valepotriates and valeric acid that have a sedative action. Valerian is thought to increase levels of an inhibitory chemical in the brain helping to dampen down over-stimulation.

Valerian is used to calm nervous, stressed and excitable horses, helping to maintain appetite.

Although feeding manufactured herbal preparations should be donewith care, there are many herbs growing naturally in pastures and hedgerows and horses such as breeding stock have free access to these. An example is hawthorn. The young shoots of the hawthorn hedges lining paddocks seem particularly appetising to horses. Hawthorn extracts contain a substance known as vitexin, which is thought to have beneficial effects on the cardiovascular system. It is also a mild diuretic. Hawthorn extracts also help to reduce the effects of stress.

Dandelion is another common herb that horses eat naturally when grazing. Dandelion or *Taraxacum officinalis* is thought of as a perennial weed. However, dandelion leaf has a diuretic action helping to remove excess water from the horse's body. It may also help to relieve liver problems. Herbs eaten fresh and whole do provide nutrients such as fibre, vitamins and minerals, in small quantities.

## VITAMIN/MINERAL SUPPLEMENTS

Broad spectrum vitamin and mineral supplements as the name suggests provide a wide range of vitamins and minerals not including salt. These may be required under certain conditions:

- Horses at pasture in winter on reduced or no concentrates
- Following viral/bacterial infections
- Overweight horses and ponies on restricted rations
- Horses and ponies on restricted pasture/turn out.

Biotin supplementation is discussed in Chapter 12.

B complex supplements are often used for horses that are post-viral or following illness/surgery or for horses that have been 'over-trained'. These supplements are given as a tonic and are very useful. B complex, particularly thiamine B1, will also help to stimulate the appetite and is excellent for post-viral horses

## ELECTROLYTES

Electrolytes or body salts refer to the minerals, sodium, potassium, chloride, calcium and magnesium. These minerals when dissolved in water become electrically charged. Sodium and chloride are contained mainly outside the cells, for example in plasma, whereas potassium is mainly contained within the cells themselves. Electrolytes are important for fluid exchange within the horse's body. They also regulate acid–base balance. Sodium, potassium, calcium and magnesium are all required to help maintain normal muscle and nerve function, obviously vital for the working horse, however sodium potassium and chloride are required in much larger quantities as they are lost in greater amounts in sweat. The kidneys help to maintain electrolyte balance by generally conserving sodium so that little is lost in urine. Sweating increases electrolyte losses drastically, particularly if prolonged, and these salts are lost from the horse's circulation and therefore body. As sodium becomes depleted, potassium steps in until it is also lost resulting in both sodium and potassium depletion. The amount and frequency of electrolyte supplementation depends upon factors including:

- Fitness
- Ambient temperature and wind factor
- Speed and terrain
- Distance of event
- Distance travelled to the event
- How well the horse drinks and eats during an endurance event.

For endurance events electrolytes should be given every 2–4 hours preferably when the horse drinks. For competition horses electrolytes should be fed after hard work and competitions.

There are many commercial electrolyte supplements available. In addition to sodium, potassium, and chloride, the supplement should contain smaller amounts of calcium and magnesium to reduce the risk of tying up and thumps. A less expensive alternative is to give the horse a mixture of 50% salt and 50% Lo-salt or Lite salt added to water at the rate of 90 g per 10 litres of water. This means 45 g salt mixed with 45 g Lo-salt or Lite salt then mixed into 10 litres of plain water. Fresh drinking water without electrolytes must also be available.

- Lite or Lo salt contains both potassium chloride and sodium chloride
- Normal salt contains sodium chloride.

A commercial electrolyte should be chosen which is salt not glucose based, however the salt based electrolytes must be introduced gradually until horses become used to the taste. Horses fed significant amounts of forage will have a good potassium intake, although sodium and chloride intakes are often low. Broodmares and youngstock should have access to a pure salt block, even in the field. Common salt should also be supplied to all working horses. If salt is added to the feed, 50g may be fed daily, rising to 100 g in warm weather. Generally most horses competing in low level competitions in cool conditions don't need electrolytes as they soon replenish losses from feed and forage and a salt block, but racehorses, showjumpers, event horses and other hard working horses such as endurance horses do need electrolyte supplementation.

## DCAB (DIETARY CATION/ANION BALANCE)

A low forage diet is likely to result in a low DCAB (dietary cation anion balance) and this can result in metabolic acidosis with consequential excretion of calcium resulting in serious muscular problems for working horses and growth related problems in young stock. A low DCAB may result in acute or chronic loss of minerals from bone and bone mineral content (BMC) is reduced. A low DCAB therefore results in Ca excretion in horses. This is not an unusual problem particularly when haylage is fed and dry matter intake is too low. Increasing forage intake, using good quality, high digestibility hay/haylage, legume chaffs and sugar beet pulp will improve the DCAB without significant adverse effects on overall dietary energy intakes.

Simply increasing the intake of over mature, low digestibility grass hay is unlikely to be successful. If haylage is being fed, the dry matter must be taken into consideration. Where forage intake is reduced feeding calcium gluconate for a few weeks to improve calcium intake until forage intake is back to normal levels (i.e. about 6 kg per day). Calcium gluconate is a highly available source of calcium. A DCAB of at least 250 mequiv/kg of dry feed helps bone retention of minerals for working and breeding horses. Check with the manufacturer.

## JOINT SUPPLEMENTS

Joint supplements are commonly fed to horses and usually contain chondroitin sulphate, glucosamine, manganese ascorbate and MSM (methylsulphonylmethane). Glucosamine may be found in several forms including sulphate and hydrochloride or as a glucosamine source.

Glucosamine sulphate is naturally made within the body from glucose and glutamine (an amino acid) and this is a slow process. Glucosamine sulphate is required to make glycosaminoglycan (GAG), which is used to lay down building blocks for new cartilage and for synovial fluid, thereby helping to heal or delay damage or lesions within the joint. Glycosaminoglycans include hyaluronan, chondroitin sulphate and keratin sulphate.

There is an injectable drug containing glycosaminoglycan, which has been approved by the relevant authorities for use in treating osteoarthritis in horses.

Results from some in vitro studies suggest that glucosamine and chondroitin sulphate may prevent the degradation of GAG and/or enhance GAG production. This does not necessarily mean that feeding in a supplement will have the same effect within the horse's joints. Other products thought to have chondroprotective or cartilage protecting effects include green-lipped muscle extract and MSM. Green lipped muscle extract is thought to contain GAG compounds and omega-3 fatty acids. MSM provides a bioavailable source of sulphur. Sulphur is part of several substances found within the joint structure.

Glucosamine may decrease the metabolic actions of insulin or may increase the risk of insulin resistance. Care should be taken when feeding glucosamine to susceptible horses, until further information become available.

## PREBIOTICS

Prebiotics are 'energy sources' that feed the beneficial microbes already present in the horse's gut. Prebiotics are not broken down in the stomach and small intestine by the horse's own enzymes and therefore naturally pass into the hindgut where they are fermented by beneficial microbes. Prebiotics are thought to enhance the immune system although research is in its early stages.

Examples of prebiotics are oligosaccharides. These are complex polysaccharides that are not broken down by digestive enzymes in the horse's small intestine. Instead they are readily broken down by beneficial bacteria in the hindgut, helping bacterial growth and therefore fibre digestion.

Fructo-oligosaccharides (FOS), for example, are used by bifidobacteria as an energy source. This helps to reduce growth of pathogenic bacteria by competitively excluding them. Mannonoligosaccharides (MOS) act differently by inhibiting pathogenic bacteria's adherence to the gut wall. Glucomannans may also help to reduce absorption of mycotoxins in horses.

## PROBIOTICS

Probiotics are 'live' microbes that are fed to horses to boost 'healthy' hindgut bacterial numbers and thereby improve fibre digestion.

Probiotic supplements provide a daily shot of live beneficial bacteria helping to top up and maintain the horse's natural eco-balance in the hindgut. Only highly resistant forms of bacteria such as lactobacillus and bifidobacterium are thought to survive transit through the stomach and small intestine before reaching the hindgut, however how many of these reach the hindgut and then colonise is open to debate. Human probiotics are coated to help this transit and further research, i.e. clinical studies with horses, is required particularly as prebiotics are now thought to be preferred.

Feeding probiotics is thought to exclude or reduce the proliferation of potentially pathogenic bacteria because the probiotics compete for food with these potentially pathogenic bacteria.

## YEAST

There are a number of yeast products available now and these are found in both compound feeds and supplements. These include yeast culture, yeast extract and dried yeast. Most of the yeast products are derived from the cultures of *Sacchromyces* spp and of these *Sacchromyces cerevisiae* is the most common.

- Dried yeast – active dried yeast should contain at least 15 billion live yeast cells per gram
- Yeast extract – the dried concentrated product resulting from ruptured *Sacchromyces cerevisiae* yeast cells
- Yeast culture – viable yeast cells and the medium upon which it has grown which is dried.

Yeast products are thought to aid fermentation and therefore fibre digestion in the hindgut of horses. Live yeast cultures are most commonly used.

Yeast cells are found within the hindgut as soon as four hours post-feeding of live yeast culture and although the cells survive there, they do not colonise and therefore yeast culture should be fed daily to maximise the beneficial digestive effects. Yeast culture is thought to increase the digestibility of the fibre (cellulose and hemicellulose) part of the diet allowing additional higher energy feeds to be fed with less risk of hindgut dysbiosis and the problems associated with this. Yeast supplemented horses had higher levels of celluloytic anaerobic bacteria (fibre digesting), lactate utilising bacteria and protozoa in the caecum, decreased gas production and reduced acetate in the colon, all of which result in improved fibre digestion and therefore increased energy supply from the hindgut. Yeast also helps to stabilise the gut microflora as it has the ability to prevent accumulation of lactic acid, helping to buffer pH thereby preventing hindgut acidosis and enabling increased uptake of key nutrients from the diet, an added bonus in the diets of performance and breeding horses.

# VITAMIN C

Under normal conditions horses do not have a requirement for extra vitamin C as this vitamin is synthesised in the liver from glucose. Research indicates that horses under stress, travelling long distances or suffering from health problems such as RAO (recurrent airway obstruction) or IAD (inflammatory airway disease) may benefit from supplemental vitamin C. The lungs sustain an environment rich in oxygen and this leaves the lung tissue susceptible to damage from free radicals. A link between bleeding from the lungs (exercise induced pulmonary haemorrhage (EIPH)) and oxidative stress has been established. Antioxidant supply is vital and these include glutathione peroxidase, alpha tocopherol and superoxide dismutase. Vitamin C supplementation may therefore be beneficial to horses suffering from respiratory disease (see Chapter 4).

# ENZYMES

Enzymes are added to the feed of other livestock to help digestion, particularly in ruminants, enzymes used include cellulases and hemicellulases that help break down fibre. It is thought that enzymes involved in fibre digestion may be useful for horses, improving digestion of poor nutritional quality forage to provide more energy. However, the research regarding enzymes in horses is in its infant stages.

## Creatine

This is used widely by human athletes but has limited use and research in horses. In humans it is believed to increase creatine phosphate in muscle for short-term high intensity exercise such as sprinting.

## DMG – dimethyl glycine

This is an intermediate substance produced when Betaine (Trimethylglycine) is metabolised.

There is some limited evidence that DMG may help reduce lactic acid build-up and thereby delay fatigue, but more research with horses is required before it can be considered for use.

## L-Carnitine

L-Carnitine is made from the essential amino acids lysine and methionine. L-Carnitine helps to transport long chain fatty acids into the mitochondria for energy production and may also regulate acetyl CoA (see Chapter 6). It is probable that horses are able to make L-Carnitine in sufficient quantities if these essential amino acids are available, i.e. it is unlikely to be deficient in performance horses on performance feeds.

---

**Summary points**

- A large number of supplements and additives are available for horses.
- Nutraceutical is a term which encompasses any supplement or additive fed for perceived health benefit.
- Before adding a supplement or additive the feeding programme should be properly evaluated to see whether or not there is an actual need.
- Overfeeding of fat-soluble vitamins and also some minerals may lead to toxicity problems. Overdosing can be fatal.
- Horses with healthy hindgut microbes are able to make their own B vitamins.
- A low forage diet is likely to result in a low DCAB (dietary cation/anion balance) resulting in metabolic acidosis.
- As many herbs contain quite potent chemicals care should be taken when feeding to pregnant mares and youngstock.
- Prebiotics are 'energy sources' that feed the beneficial hindgut microbes.
- B complex vitamins are useful for post-viral horses.
- Vitamin C supplementation may be beneficial to horses suffering from respiratory disease.

---

# Formulating a Ration

Calculating rations for horses can be daunting, but this will enable horse owners to achieve a balanced feeding programme, which will help to maintain health and performance of horses. To formulate a ration the current nutrient requirements for horses are required. In the following examples the energy, protein and lysine requirements are calculated using NRC 2007 data.

## NUTRIENT REQUIREMENTS

Nutrient requirements of horses are published by the NRC National Research Council (USA) the latest edition being the 6th revised edition in 2007. The horse's nutrient requirements vary depending on factors such as activity and stage of life cycle. Generally, nutrient requirements are shown according to the following classifications:

- Maintenance
- Work
- Growth
- Gestation/pregnancy
- Lactation.

For example, a maintenance ration is designed for a mature, idle horse to maintain weight and body condition under normal climate conditions. Non-working adult horses and ponies can be maintained on high quality forages without concentrate feeds, although the pasture and/ or forage may not be balanced for micronutrients, particularly minerals, and these may need to be supplemented.

The horse's requirement for energy increases 25%, 50% and 100% as the work level increases from light, to moderate, to heavy. Growing, breeding and working/competing horses will need concentrate supplementation to meet the additional nutrient requirements. During pregnancy, the mare's requirement for protein, minerals and vitamins increases. As pregnancy moves through the later stages the mare's need for energy increases up to 20%. Lactation also means additional requirements for protein, minerals and vitamins and particularly energy as lactation places enormous metabolic stress on mares.

Stressful conditions associated with a horse's environment may also affect the nutrient requirements. Changes in temperature, moisture and humidity as well as poor grazing, overstocking, travel, competing and overwork are a few examples of situations that can lead to stress. These and other factors can alter the horse's need for various nutrients and should be taken into account.

Horses are naturally trickle feeding herbivores and therefore rations must be based on forage for mature horses. When calculating rations the requirements assume feed intakes of 2.5% BW (bodyweight) for horses in hard work, lactating mares and growing youngstock, 2.25% BW for medium work and 2% BW for all others. For example, a horse in hard work should eat about 2.5% of its body weight in feed each day. A mature 500 kg horse will therefore eat around 12.5 kg DM (dry matter) each day. (For a 1000 lb horse this is roughly 25 lb.) Ideally, horses should consume a minimum of 1.0% of the body weight as forage each day and, as a general rule, forage should comprise at least 50% of the total weight of daily feed. Concentrates, fat, supplemental protein, vitamins and minerals are important, but should make up a much smaller portion of the ration and only when required. The nutrient requirements for all classes of horses are given in Appendix 1.

## RATION FORMULATION

This process does require some basic calculations. Most horse owners do not have access to complicated computer programs that are able to instantly calculate all the requirements for a given weight and category of horse. Computer programs are the most accurate method of formulating rations, but often adjustments from knowledgeable nutritionists are still needed. Compound feeds have already been formulated and nutritionally balanced to take out this guess work and will provide all nutrients required for a given workload, if fed at the recommended rate. A horse needs approximately 40 different nutrients in the diet, trying to balance all these without a computer is extremely difficult and time consuming. Fortunately most of these nutrients are provided by rations with reasonable levels of good quality forage. The nutrients where deficiencies may more often occur are:

- Digestible energy
- Crude protein (amino acid profile should be good)
- Calcium
- Phosphorus
- Vitamin A
- Vitamin E (working horses and breeding stock)
- Copper (breeding stock)
- Selenium.

Here we will assess energy, protein, lysine (an important essential amino acid) Ca and P requirements for two different types of horse.

Before calculating a ration some important information is needed such as:

- How much does the horse weigh?
- What condition is the horse?
- How much work is the horse doing, if any?
- Is the horse growing?
- Is the mare pregnant or lactating?
- Nutrient content of the forage
- Which feeds are available, straights/compounds?

## Step 1 – Assessment of bodyweight

Bodyweight may be calculated by several means:

- Portable weighbridge
- Bodyweight tape as supplied by feed companies
- Calculation from a formula.

The portable weighbridge is the most accurate and these are often found in larger yards and studs. Bodyweight tapes are approximately 90% accurate and probably the calculation below would be preferred.

The horse's bodyweight may also be calculated from the following formulae which use the horse's heart girth measurement and length as measured with a tape measure from point of shoulder to point of buttock (Figure 10.1).

$$\text{Bodyweight} (\text{kg}) = \frac{\text{Heart girth} (\text{cm})^2 \times \text{Length} (\text{cm})}{11,880}$$

$$\text{Bodyweight} (\text{lbs}) = \frac{\text{Heart girth} (\text{inches})^2 \times \text{Length} (\text{inches})}{330}$$

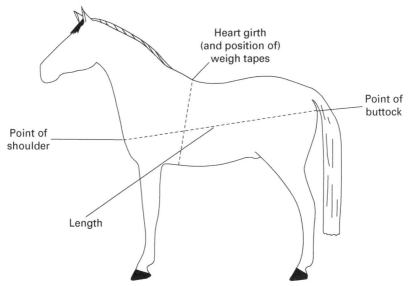

**Figure 10.1** Calculation of bodyweight from measurements.

For foals up to 6 weeks of age use the following

$$\text{Bodyweight in kg} = \frac{\text{Heart girth (cm)} - 63.7}{0.38}$$

$$\text{Bodyweight in lb} = \frac{\text{Heart girth (inches)} - 25.1}{0.07}$$

Once the bodyweight is ascertained, the total dry matter intake per day may be calculated.

## Step 2 – Calculation of dry matter intake

As discussed earlier this will depend upon the work level and condition of the horse. As a general rule horses need from 1.5% to 2.5% of bodyweight per day depending upon the individual needs. Horses in hard work or lactating mares will need 2.5% of bodyweight per day whereas a very overweight horse or pony may need the minimum of 1.5% per day. For horses at maintenance or in light work, 2% BW should be used. In the following calculations two horses are used as examples, Wilfred and Harvey.

**Wilfred** (Figure 10.2) – overweight mature cob, bodyweight 550 kg, laid back type (light work). DM intake may be calculated as follows:

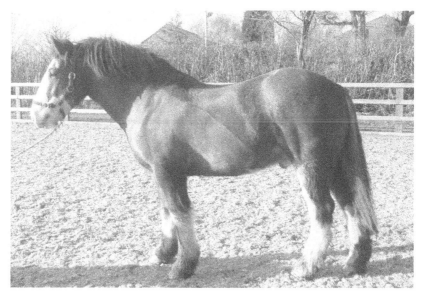

**Figure 10.2**  Wilfred – mature cob, tendency to be overweight (Courtesy of Dr E. Church).

2.0% intake = 2.0 divided by $100 \times 550 = 11$ kg DM/day

2.5% intake = 2.5 divided by $100 \times 550 = 12.38$ kg DM/day

(would provide too much energy increasing weight gain)

**Harvey** (Figure 10.3) – TB cross, mature competition horse, nervous type (hard work) bodyweight 525 kg. DM Intake is as follows:

2.5% intake = 2.5 divided by $100 \times 525 = 13.13$ kg DM/day

1.5% intake = 1.5 divided by $100 \times 525 = 7.88$ kg/day

(this would not provide enough energy to meet requirements leading to weight loss)

This formula works well for mature horses but not for foals and weanlings:

- DM Intake for foals up to 6 months is about 0.5–0.75% BW while nursing
- DM Intake for weanlings is up to 3.5% BW per day.

## Step 3 – Forage to concentrate ratio

As previously mentioned, mature horses should be fed a minimum of 1% BW or 50% of the total ration as forage, whichever is the greater. This includes pasture hay/haylage and any chaff products or other

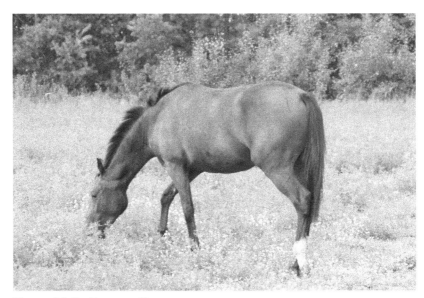

**Figure 10.3** Harvey – TB cross, nervous type.

**Table 10.1** Forage to concentrate ratios.

|  | %Forage | %Concentrates |
| --- | --- | --- |
| Maintenance/light work | 80–100 | 0–20 |
| Medium work | 60 | 40 |
| Hard work | 50 | 50 |
| Pregnant mare last 3 months | 70 | 30 |
| Lactating mare | 50 | 50 |
| Foal nursing | 30 | 70 |
| Weanling | 50 | 50 |
| Yearling | 60 | 40 |

forage. Foals and yearlings may need more concentrates than forage as the gut is not fully able to digest fibre. Forage to concentrate ratios are given in Table 10.1.

Wilfred in light work would therefore need 80% forage and 20% concentrates.

Harvey in hard work would need 50% forage and 50% concentrates.

It is important to remember that different feedstuffs have different dry matter values. DM is the remainder after water has been removed. The DM values for typical horse feeds are shown in Table 10.2.

**Table 10.2** Typical DM content of horse feeds.

|  | Dry matter % | Water content % |
|---|---|---|
| Cereal straights oats, barley, maize, bran. | 87 | 13 |
| Compound feeds cubes, coarse mixes | 85–90 | 10–15 |
| Hay | 86–90 | 10–14 |
| Haylage | 60–75 | 25–40 |
| Pasture spring | 20 | 80 |
| Pasture winter | 30 | 70 |

There is little information regarding voluntary dry matter intake (VDMI) of horses at pasture, as this has proved difficult to measure in practice.

Estimates of VDMI of pasture generally range from 1.5% to 3.0% BW per day with the highest intakes in lactating mares. It is thought the average horse would consume 2% VDMI per day and so this value is used as a rule of thumb.

Some horses at maintenance or in light work on good quality pasture and or hay/haylage might meet all their energy and protein needs without the need for extra concentrate feeds supplying further energy and protein. However, a pasture balancer or broad spectrum vitamin and mineral supplement may still be required particularly in the winter months to make up any micronutrient deficiencies in the pasture.

The actual nutrient content of forage can only be achieved by nutrient analysis. Conserved forage such as hay or haylage should be purchased with at least a basic analysis, although this is not always possible. If not, then the average values as listed in Appendix 2 or NRC (National Research Council 6th revised edition in 2007) should be used instead. This also applies to straight cereals and fortunately these do not vary very much from year to year. Compound feeds such as cubes and mixes must supply a basic analysis by law known as the statutory statement, which is shown on the feed tag or label (see Chapter 8). Any further information required may be obtained from the feed manufacturer.

## Step 4 – Energy calculations

Energy requirements are given as Mcal DE or MJ DE per day (megacalories or megajoules digestible energy).

To convert Mcal to MJ simply multiply by 4.184 or 4.2. Requirements are listed as both in Appendices 1 and 2. In USA Mcals tend to be used whereas in the UK MJ are the unit of choice.

**Table 10.3**   Energy values for maintenance $E_m$ (NRC 2007).

| Bodyweight kg | Minimum 0.0303 Mcal/kg BW | Average 0.0333 Mcal/kg BW | Elevated 0.0363 Mcal/kg BW | NRC 1989 |
|---|---|---|---|---|
| 200 | 6.1 | 6.7 | 7.3 | 7.4 |
| 500 | 15.2 | 16.7 | 18.2 | 16.4 |
| 600 | 18.2 | 20.0 | 21.8 | 19.4 |

## Energy for maintenance

NRC 2007 has adjusted energy requirements for maintenance according to different types of horses. There are now three calculations giving minimum, average and elevated values:

- Minimum – idle horses, stabled/box rest limited turnout
- Average – daily turnout, average temperament
- Elevated – daily turnout, working, lactating, growing, nervous types.

1. **Wilfred – cob 550 kg**
   As this cob is overweight and quite laid back the minimum value for maintenance should be used.
      Energy for maintenance ($E_m$) is therefore calculated as follows

   $0.303 \times 550 = 16.6$ Mcal/day

   $16.6 \times 4.184 = 69.5$ MJ/day

   So Wilfred requires 69.5 MJ/day energy for maintenance.

2. **Harvey – 525 kg competition horse**
   Assuming this horse is in hard work and a nervous type, the elevated energy for maintenance $E_m$ is preferred.

   $0.0363 \times 525 = 19.1$ Mcal/day

   $19.1 \times 4.184 = 79.9$ MJ/day

   So Harvey requires 79.9 MJ/day energy for maintenance.
   When horses are also working we can calculate the energy needed for both maintenance and work (Table 10.4).

*For horses with minimum maintenance requirements use 0.0303 and if elevated use 0.0363 as discussed above.*

1. Wilfred – 550 kg cob
   We have calculated Wilfred needs 69.5 MJ/day for maintenance; if he is also working we can calculate new totals to include the energy

**Table 10.4**  Energy requirements for work.

| Work level | Heart rate | Type of work (examples) | DE Mcal/day For minimum maintenance requirement | DE Mcal/day For elevated maintenance requirement | DE Mcal/day For elevated maintenance requirement |
|---|---|---|---|---|---|
| Light | 80 beats/min | Early training schooling Recreational riding, hacking | $(0.0303\,BW) \times 1.2$ | $(0.0333\,BW) \times 1.2$ | $(0.0363\,BW) \times 1.2$ |
| Medium | 90 beats/min | Pleasure ride Mid training, Low level eventing | $(0.0303\,BW) \times 1.4$ | $(0.0333\,BW) \times 1.4$ | $(0.0363\,BW) \times 1.4$ |
| Hard | 110 beats/min | Canter/gallop Hard schooling | $(0.0303\,BW) \times 1.6$ | $(0.0333\,BW) \times 1.6$ | $(0.0363\,BW) \times 1.6$ |

he also requires for working from Table 10.4 (Wilfred has **minimum** $E_m$ requirements).

Light work $= (0.0303 \times 550) \times 1.2 = 20$ Mcal/day

$20 \times 4.184 = 83.7$ MJ/day

Medium work $= (0.0303 \times 550) \times 1.4 = 23.3$ Mcal/day

$23.3 \times 4.184 = 97.5$ MJ/day

Wilfred is overweight so will not be up to hard work, but if he were the calculation would be as follows:

Hard work $= (0.0303 \times 550) \times 1.6 = 26.6$ Mcal/day

$26.6 \times 4.184 = 111.3$ MJ/day

2. We can now work out Harvey's energy needs if working.
   Harvey 525 kg competition horse
   (Harvey has **elevated** $E_m$ requirements)

   Light work $=(0.0363 \times 525) \times 1.2 = 22.9$ Mcal/day

   $22.9 \times 4.184 = 95.8$ MJ/day

   Medium work $= (0.0363 \times 525) \times 1.4 = 26.7$ Mcal/day

   $26.7 \times 4.184 = 111.7$ MJ/day

   Hard work $= (0.0363 \times 525) \times 1.6 = 30.5$ Mcal/day

   $30.5 \times 4.184 = 127.6$ MJ/day

   A summary of Wilfred's and Harvey's energy requirements is shown in Table 10.5.

**Table 10.5**  Energy requirements MJ/day.

|  | Maintenance | Light work | Medium work | Hard work |
|---|---|---|---|---|
| Wilfred 550 kg | 69.5 | 83.7 | 97.5 | 111.3 |
| Harvey 525 kg | 79.9 | 95.8 | 111.7 | 127.6 |

**Table 10.6**  Extra protein requirements for work.

|  | Maintenance | Light work | Medium work | Hard work |
|---|---|---|---|---|
| Wilfred 550 kg | 594 g | +49 g | +97.4 g | +146.3 g |
| Harvey 525 kg | 756 g | +46.7 g | +93 g | +139.6 g |

# Step 5 – Crude protein calculations

Crude protein intake is calculated from the energy requirements for all horses except for lactating mares. The essential amino acid lysine requirement may then be calculated from the crude protein.

The crude protein for maintenance can be calculated as follows:

- Minimum – BW × 1.08 g CP/kg BW/day
- Average – BW × 1.26 g CP/kg BW/day
- Elevated – BW × 1.44 g CP/kg BW/day.

From these formulae we can work out Wilfred and Harvey's protein requirements for maintenance

Wilfred – Minimum – 550 × 1.08 = 594 g CP/day

Harvey – Elevated – 525 × 1.44 = 756 g CP/day

Then we can add the extra protein required for different work levels. Working horses need some additional protein to replace nitrogen losses from sweat and building additional muscle. Although these increases are relatively small see Table 10.6.

Extra crude protein requirements for work are as follows:

- Light work – BW × 0.089 g CP/kg BW/day
- Medium work – BW × 0.177 g CP/kg BW/day
- Hard work – BW × 0.266 g CP/kg BW/day.

These formulae can be used to calculate the extra protein required for work.

So Wilfred in light work would need 594 + 49 = 643 g protein/day

Harvey in hard work would need 756 + 139.6 = 895.6 g protein/day

## Step 6 – Lysine requirements

Lysine can be calculated from the daily crude protein.

Lysine g/day = 4.3 % of the crude protein requirement, therefore:

Wilfred in light work would need 27.6 g lysine per day

Harvey in hard work would need 38.5 g lysine per day

## Step 7 – Calcium can be calculated from the following equations

Maintenance – 0.04 g Ca/kg BW

Light exercise – 0.06 g Ca/kg BW

Med/hard exercise – 0.07 g Ca/kg BW

Therefore

Wilfred, light exercise = 550 × 0.06 = 33 g Ca

Harvey hard work = 525 × 0.07 = 36.8 g Ca

## Step 8 – Phosphorus can be calculated from the following equations

Maintenance – 0.04 g P/kg BW

Light exercise – 0.036 g P/kg BW

Med/Hard exercise – 0.058 g P/kg BW

Therefore

Wilfred, light exercise = 550 × 0.036 = 19.8 g P

Harvey hard work = 525 × 0.058 = 30.5 g P

Now the daily amounts of these major nutrients are known the ration can be assessed to check if it is meeting these requirements. In other words, convert these figures into a practical ration. For ease we will take the previous examples of Wilfred and Harvey as previously calculated and assume Wilfred is in light work and Harvey is in hard work (Table 10.7).

Wilfred – bodyweight 550 kg, overweight mature cob, laid back type (light work)

**Table 10.7**   Table summaries of the total daily nutrients required as calculated.

|  | Energy | Protein | Lysine | Ca | P |
|---|---|---|---|---|---|
| Wilfred 550 kg Light work | 83.7 MJ | 643 g | 27.6 g | 33 g | 19.8 g |
| Harvey 525 kg Hard work | 127.6 MJ | 895.6 g | 38.5 g | 36.8 g | 30.5 g |

**Table 10.8**

|  | Wilfred Total | Wilfred From hay 80% | Wilfred From conc. 20% | Harvey Total | Harvey From hay 50% | Harvey From conc. 50% |
|---|---|---|---|---|---|---|
| DE MJ/day | 83.7 | 66.7 | 17 | 127.6 | 63.8 | 63.8 |
| CP g/day | 643 | 500 | 143 | 900 | 450 | 450 |
| Lysine g/day | 27.6 | 22.1 | 5.5 | 38.5 | 19.25 | 19.25 |

Previously worked out information includes the daily DM intake and forage to concentrate ratios as follows

2.0% intake = 2.0 divided by $100 \times 550 = 11$ kg DM feed/day

Wilfred in light work would therefore be 80% forage and 20% concentrates

$0.8 \times 11 = 8.8$ kg forage/DM/day

$0.2 \times 11 = 2.2$ kg concentrates/DM/day

Harvey – bodyweight 525 kg, TB type, mature competition horse, nervous type (hard work)

2.5% intake = 2.5 divided by $100 \times 525 = 13.13$ kg DM/day

Harvey in hard work would need 50% forage and 50% concentrates

$0.5 = 13.13 = 6.56$ kg forage/DM/day

$0.5 \times 13.13 = 6.56$ kg forage/DM/day

Table 10.8 shows the daily nutrient requirements from hay and forage for both horses as previously calculated.

Table 10.9 gives average figures for example feeds for Wilfred and Harvey.

**Table 10.9** Compound feeds and forage.

| | Racehorse cubes | Horse & pony cubes | Performance mix | Balancer | Average hay | Good hay | Average haylage |
|---|---|---|---|---|---|---|---|
| Dry matter % | 90 | 90 | 88 | 90 | 88 | 88 | 65 |
| DE MJ/kg | 13 | 10 | 12 | 11 | 8 | 9.5 | 9.5 |
| CP% | 14 | 10 | 12 | 20 | 7 | 8 | 9 |
| Starch % | 23 | 8 | 16.5 | 16 | – | – | – |
| Lysine % | 0.55 | 0.55 | 0.6 | 1.05 | 0.5 | 0.7 | 0.7 |
| Calcium % | 1.5 | 1.0 | 1.5 | 2.5 | 0.7 | 0.9 | 0.9 |
| Phosphorus % | 0.45 | 0.45 | 0.5 | 1.0 | 0.3 | 0.4 | 0.4 |
| Vit E IU/kg | 200 | 150 | 150 | 1200 | – | – | – |

## A – Daily digestible energy intake (MJ/day)

### Wilfred (DMI – 11 kg)

Wilfred needs 66.7 MJ energy from average hay, which contains 8 MJ/kg DM

So 66.7/8 = 8.34 kg hay will therefore provide 66.7 MJ DE.
Adjust for **dry matter** from **as fed**
Hay contains 88% DM therefore

8.34/0.88 = 9.5 kg hay

Remaining energy from concentrates is 17 MJ. In this case horse and pony cubes which contain 9 MJ/kg DM.

17/9 = 1.8 kg cubes

Adjust for dry matter from as fed
Cubes contain 90% DM therefore

1.8/0.9 = 2 kg cubes

According to Wilfred's bodyweight, calculation of total daily DM Intake was 11 kg (2.0% BW for 550 kg horse). The total above is 11.5 kg total feed (DM), which is just above and could be adjusted downwards to help Wilfred lose weight slowly if required, i.e. it will provide less energy per day.

### Harvey (DMI –13.13 kg)

Needs 63.8 MJ energy from good hay which contains 9.5 MJ/kg DM
So 63.8/9.5 = 6.71 kg hay will therefore provide 63.8 MJ DE.
Adjust for **dry matter** from **as fed**
Hay contains 88% DM therefore

6.71/0.88 = 7.6 kg hay

(**NB** If haylage is fed, 6.71 kg haylage DM would provide the 63.8 MJ required, however the adjustment for dry matter is very important. This is a common misconception as when haylage is fed, more haylage than hay is required, not less.

6.71/0.65(DM%) = 10.3 kg haylage would need to be fed to take into account the additional water in haylage.)

Remaining energy from concentrates is 17 MJ. In this case performance mix which contains 12 MJ/kg DM.

63.8/12 = 5.31 kg performance mix

Adjust for **dry matter** from **as fed**
This mix contains 88% DM therefore

5.31/0.88 = 6 kg performance mix

According to Harvey's bodyweight, calculation of total daily DM Intake was 13.13 kg (2.5% BW for 550 kg horse). The total above is 13.6 kg total feed (DM) which is just above the BW calculation This slight increase is required if Harvey is to maintain condition while working at this level.

## B – Daily crude protein (g/day)

Crude protein may be calculated by using the grids shown in Tables 10.10 (Wilfred) and 10.11 (Harvey).

Total % CP in Wilfred's ration = 0.865/11.5 × 100 = 7.5%

NRC CP requirements for Wilfred (see Table 10.11) = 643 g/day so this ration exceeds by 222 g/day or 34%. This is not unusual, as most

**Table 10.10**  Crude protein – Wilfred.

| Average hay at 7% CP | 9.5 kg | 7% | 665 g protein |
|---|---|---|---|
| H&P cubes at 10% CP | 2 kg | 10% | 200 g protein |
|  | 11.5 kg |  | 865 g total protein |
|  | (11,500 g) |  |  |

**Table 10.11**  Crude protein – Harvey.

| Good hay at 9% CP | 7.6 kg | 8% | 608 g protein |
|---|---|---|---|
| Performance mix at 13% CP | 6.0 kg | 13% | 780 g protein |
|  | 13.6 kg |  | 1388 g total protein |
|  | (13,600 g) |  |  |

rations containing high amounts of forage will exceed protein requirements.

Total % CP in Harvey's ration $= 1388/13,600 \times 100 = 10.2\%$

NRC CP requirements for Harvey (see Table 10.11) $= 900\,g/day$ so this ration exceeds by $488\,g$ /day or 54%. Again this is not unusual as most rations containing high amounts of forage will exceed protein requirements and in this case is combined with higher protein performance mix. Alfalfa hay would greatly exceed the protein requirements.

## C – Daily lysine (g/day)

Lysine may be calculated as shown in Table 10.12.

Total lysine % in Wilfred's ration $= 58.5/11,500 \times 100 = 0.5\%$

NRC lysine requirements for Wilfred (see Table 10.11) $= 27.6\,g/day$ so this ration exceeds by $32\,g/day$ or 54%. Again this is not unusual, as most rations containing high amounts of forage will exceed lysine requirements.

Total lysine % in Harvey's ration $= 89.2/13,600 \times 100 = 0.65\%$

NRC lysine requirements for Harvey (see Table 10.11) $= 38.5\,g/day$ so this ration exceeds by $50\,g$ /day or 56%. This is not unusual as most rations containing high amounts of forage will exceed lysine requirements and in this case is combined with higher protein and therefore lysine performance mix. Alfalfa hay would greatly exceed the lysine requirements.

   Similar calculations to those above can then be carried out for calcium and phosphorus.

**Table 10.12**   Lysine – Wilfred.

| | | | |
|---|---|---|---|
| Average hay at 0.5% Lys | 9.5 kg | 0.5% | 47.5 g lysine |
| H&P cubes at 0.55% Lys | 2 kg | 0.55% | 11.0 g lysine |
| | 11.5 kg | | 58.5 g total lysine |
| | (11,500g) | | |

**Table 10.13**   Lysine – Harvey.

| | | | |
|---|---|---|---|
| Good hay at 0.7% Lys | 7.6 kg | 0.7% | 53.2 g lysine |
| Performance mix at 0.6% Lys | 6.0 kg | 0.6% | 36 g lysine |
| | 13.6 kg | | 89.2 g total lysine |
| | (13,600 g) | | |

## SUMMARY

For both Wilfred and Harvey the macronutrient requirements have been calculated from NRC 2007 data and have been met and mostly exceeded. Energy requirements are the most important to maintain condition and energy for work. For Wilfred, reducing energy intake slightly will help him to lose excess weight over time.

In addition Wilfred's intake of horse and pony cubes is low compared with the recommended feeding levels and so an additional broad spectrum vitamin and mineral supplement should be supplied particularly in the winter months. Alternatively, the horse and pony cubes could be replaced by a forage balancer most of which are fed at the rate of 500 g to 1 kg per day with the hay. If Wilfred is out at pasture the hay intake should be reduced accordingly in the summer months, probably to zero, whereas in winter the hay will be required in greater amounts.

Harvey's performance mix should contain the micronutrients to meet requirements at this level of concentrate feed intake. If out at pasture during the day the hay intake can be reduced.

Bodyweight should be monitored to check the horse's energy requirements are being met. If a horse needs to lose condition, reducing the feed intake slightly will help it to slowly lose excess weight particularly if combined with exercise. If more condition is required the horse's daily energy intake should be increased. Condition scoring is an excellent tool for horse owners to assess true condition of the horse.

For all horses minor adjustments will probably be required depending upon the individual. For hungry horses, concentrates should be reduced and forage increased. For horses in hard work with poor appetites forage may need to be reduced to the minimum level and concentrates increased to give a higher energy density.

## CONDITION SCORE

Condition score simply assesses visually and by gentle touch the amount of body fat covering particular points of the horse's skeleton, for example the point of hips, buttocks, spine, ribs, and neck. Although some of these areas may also be heavily muscled, such as the hindquarters and tail head, with a little practice and light prodding of the area, the difference between muscle and fat can easily be ascertained. Condition scoring does not take into account gut fill (or fat underbellies) therefore making it an accurate method of assessing and monitoring the horse's condition. There are several conditioning scoring systems including one for donkeys – some use a 9 point scale but the one most commonly used by vets and nutritionists is the 5 point scale.

Each horse is assigned a score from 0 to 5, zero being very poor or emaciated and five being obese. Figure 10.4 shows an overweight horse with a condition score of 4/5 whereas Figure 10.5 shows an underweight horse with a condition score of 0/5.

The areas of assessment are as follows: neck, withers, shoulder, ribs, backbone, tail head, point of hips, point of buttocks and inner thighs.

Starting at the head, the horse should be carefully appraised by look and feel, and given a score to each area from 0 to 5 as listed above. The average score is then taken of all the points measured to give an overall condition score for the horse.

This will take into account conformational differences such as through the croup and long and short backs.

Table 10.14 gives all the criteria required to allocate a condition score to horses. Horses should be standing in a well lit area while being assessed. Figure 10.6 shows the appearance over the pelvic area.

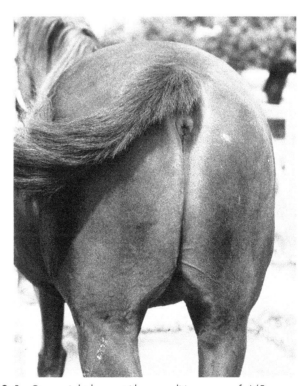

**Figure 10.4**  Overweight horse with a condition score of 4/5.

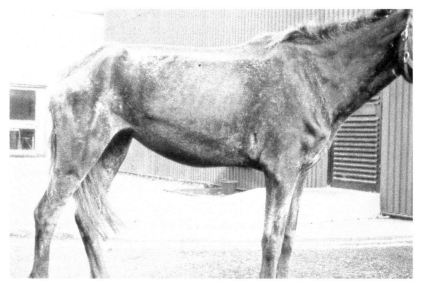

**Figure 10.5** Severely underweight horse, condition score 0. This figure was published in *Diseases and Disorders of the Horse*, Knottenbelt and Pascoe. Copyright: Elsevier (1994).

**Table 10.14** Condition scoring table.

| Condition score | Pelvis | Back and ribs | Base of neck |
|---|---|---|---|
| 0 | Deep cavity under tail and either side of croup. Pelvis angular. No detectable fatty tissue between skin and bone | Processes of vertebrae 'sharply pointed' to touch, Skin drawn tightly over ribs | Ewe neck, very narrow and slack at base |
| 1 | Pelvis and croup well defined, no fat, but skin supple. Poverty lines visible and deep depression under tail | Ribs and backbone clearly defined but skin slack over the bones | Ewe neck, narrow and slack at base |
| 2 | Croup well defines but some fat under skin. Pelvis easily felt, slight depression under tail | Backbone just covered by fat, individual vertebral processes not visible but easily felt on pressure. Ribs just visible | Narrow but firm |
| 3 | Whole pelvic region rounded, not angular and no gutter along croup. Skin smooth and supple and pelvis easily felt | Backbone and ribs well covered and only felt on firm pressure. Gutter along backbone | Narrow but with no crest (except stallions) |
| 4 | Pelvis buried in fat and only felt on firm pressure. Gutter over croup | Backbone and ribs well covered and only felt on firm pressure. Gutter along backbone | Wide and firm with folds of fat. Slight crest even on mares |
| 5 | Pelvis buried in fat and cannot be felt. Clear deep gutter over croup to base of dock. Skin stretched | Back looks flat with deep gutter along backbone Ribs buried and cannot be felt | Very wide and firm. Marked crest |

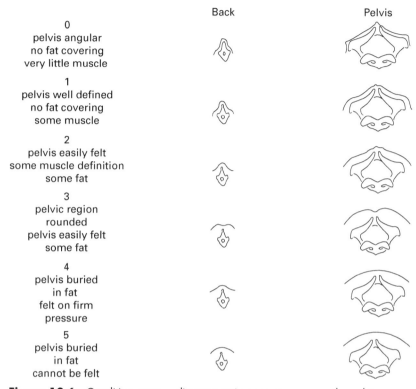

                                    Back                    Pelvis

0
pelvis angular
no fat covering
very little muscle

1
pelvis well defined
no fat covering
some muscle

2
pelvis easily felt
some muscle definition
some fat

3
pelvic region
rounded
pelvis easily felt
some fat

4
pelvis buried
in fat
felt on firm
pressure

5
pelvis buried
in fat
cannot be felt

**Figure 10.6**   Condition score – diagrammatic appearance over the pelvic area.

---

**Summary points**

- Calculating rations of horses can be daunting, but this will help to achieve a balanced feeding programme.
- The horse's nutrient requirements vary depending on factors such as activity and stage of life cycle.
- NRC 2007 has adjusted energy requirements for maintenance according to different types of horses. There are now three calculations giving minimum, average and elevated values.
- Bodyweight should be monitored to check the horse's energy requirements are being met.
- Condition score simply assesses visually and by gentle touch the amount and depth of body fat covering.
- Each horse is assigned a score from 0 to 5, zero being very poor or emaciated and five being obese.

# Feeding Different Types of Horses

All horses apart from young foals must have good quality forage first and foremost in the diet. This should then be nutritionally balanced for any further nutrients that may be required, usually energy and micronutrients. Fibre is a vital part of the equine diet and is not just a "filler".

## Breeding stock

### Barren mares

Barren mares should be kept in good condition for future breeding and fed a maintenance diet (energy wise) with plenty of quality forage. In addition a stud formulation vitamin and mineral supplement or a stud balancer is important so that all micronutrients are available following conception and during early embryonic and foetal development.

### Pregnant mares

Traditionally pregnant mares are fed as for maintenance from early to mid-pregnancy. This is then increased for the last three months of pregnancy. New research into developmental orthopaedic disease (DOD) shows that balanced nutrition of the mare throughout pregnancy plays a significant role in reducing the incidence of DOD in foals.

Mares should be fed a balanced ration from day one of pregnancy. Low energy, nutritionally formulated stud balancers are ideal for this purpose and can be fed alongside good quality forage. This is a more natural ration as it is low in starch and relies more on fibre from forage to meet energy needs and helps to maintain the health of the digestive tract. Mares requiring more condition may be fed stud cubes.

Pregnant mares should be kept in good condition all year round (3/4). Mares with a condition score of less than 2 are more likely to skip a breeding season whereas very overweight mares may have problems foaling.

Broodmares fed large grain based meals to increase condition prior to foaling or to influence imminent milk production, are more likely to develop significant digestive problems such as colic and laminitis. Mares fed a high fibre and oil ration balanced with important minerals vitamins and amino acids are less likely to suffer from metabolic or digestive disorders at this important time.

Feeding higher levels of vitamin E for one month prior to and one month after foaling appears to improve both colostrum and blood levels of this important vitamin. Enhanced levels of the immunoglobulins, IgG, IgM and IgA in colostrum were found. Feeding a stud cube with around 400 IU/kg vitE of feed is therefore recommended. Vitamin E is closely linked to reproductive efficiency in mares but more research is required.

Following birth, mares should be fed a small amount of warm mash of the normal feed as parturition demands a huge amount of energy from the mare. (Figure 11.1).

Further work regarding essential fatty acids has shown that these may have excellent health benefits to mares as omega 3 fatty acids are often in short supply in winter pasture. Important essential omega 3

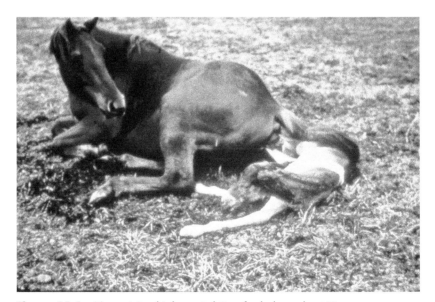

**Figure 11.1**  Mare giving birth, a vital time for balanced nutrition.

fattyacids are α-linolenic acid (ALA), eicosapentaenoic acid (EPA), and docosahexaenoic acid (DHA). These fatty acids are essential for normal growth and development of the foetus.

## Lactating mares

A typical thoroughbred lactating mare will produce an astonishing 11–14 kg milk per day for the first three months. This amount will decrease to about 8 kg per day by five months. This represents approximately 450 gallons over a 150 day period, placing a huge nutrient drain on the mare. The lactating mare has increased requirements for energy water, protein, calcium and phosphorus in particular to produce milk. A deficiency in any of these nutrients is unlikely to affect the quality of milk produced, but will cause the mare to use up her own mineral stores causing deficiencies in the mare and foal and possible problems with rebreeding.

Research has shown when lactating mares are fed concentrates based upon fat/oil and fibre as compared with starch based cereal concentrates, milk composition is affected in ways that help to improve the health of suckling foals. Levels of alpha linolenic acid (an essential fatty acid) in milk are improved and this in turn may lead to a reduction in gastric ulcers in foals. Higher colostrum levels of IgG were also found. Mares fed fibre and fat diets should also be fed a stud formulation vitamin and mineral supplement or low calorie stud balancer which contains a nutritional balance of quality amino acids, vitamins and minerals. If a higher calorie concentrate feed is preferred, particularly in the first three months when energy requirements are highest, stud cubes are likely to be lower in starch than stud mixes. Oil can then be added which helps to reduce the GI of the feed and increase the calories.

Researchers have shown there is no benefit to supplementing with higher levels of zinc, copper and iron beyond requirement levels. Mares may be prepared for weaning by feeding plenty of top quality forage, with alfalfa/beet pulp and oil and a stud balancer or stud supplement supplying vitamins, minerals and quality amino acids. Further trials showed that lactating mares need an adequate intake of the essential amino acid methionine, selenium and iodine for renewed fertility and foetal development. This is obviously important for lactating mares that are rebred in the same season. Again these should be supplied adequately in the concentrate ration.

The quantity of stud feed required will depend upon the concentrate feed chosen, but heavily lactating mares may need as much as 1.5% of their bodyweight as concentrates per day. For a typical 500 kg TB mare this equates to as much 7.5 kg (16.5 lb) stud cubes per day split between four feeds (balancers will be fed at a much lower rate and feeding instructions should be closely followed). The amount will depend upon the quality and intake of forage/pasture. Most mares (apart from TB early foalers) will have access to spring and summer pasture of good quality and this will significantly reduce the amount of high energy concentrates required, but stub balancers may still be beneficial to make up any possible mineral deficiencies in pasture.

## Foals

Foals grow at extremely fast rates particularly during the first six months of life. Daily gains of over 1 kg during the suckling phase until weaning at six months are very common. A typical TB foal may drink 25% of their bodyweight per day as milk.

Once born, the foal is dependent upon the dam's milk supply during the first few weeks of life. Milk is the main source of nutrition until the foal reaches 4–5 months of age. Foals are born with a monogastric digestive tract (similar to humans) and do not have the capacity at this stage to digest forage. This develops over the next 3–6 months. Research has shown that mares produce milk at the rate of approximately 3–4% of their bodyweight for the first twelve weeks of lactation and this then falls to 2% until weaning. Mare's milk has also been the subject of considerable investigation and has been found to contain low levels of certain minerals such as iron, copper and zinc, which are important for bone growth and development. If pasture is also low in these minerals, then the foal will rapidly use up its own body reserves during this vital growth phase and will need supplementary feeding with a stud balancer, i.e. a foal creep feed.

Some foals will eat the dam's droppings (coprophagy) up to approximately 2 months age. This is thought to be normal, helping to populate the hindgut with microbes.

## Orphan foals

A good foster mare is the ideal solution but this is not always possible. There are numerous mare's milk replacers available and most are powders, which are mixed with water before use. Cow's milk may also be used if mixed with skimmed milk half and half, as cow's milk alone is too rich. The manufacturer's mixing instructions should be followed accurately. The initial concern with a newly orphaned foal (or any foal for that matter) from birth is that it receives colostrum, as this offers some protection from disease. Ideally the foal should be given 250 ml colostrum hourly for six hours after birth. The foal should then have its antibody status checked at 12–36 hours to check that passive transfer has occurred, i.e. an antibody concentration of IgG 4–8 g/l has been achieved. If the foal has not received enough colostrum, it may be given a blood plasma transfer by the vet, if IgG is less than 4 g/l.

If a foster mare is not available, then the foal will need hand rearing by bottle. Milk should be given at a rate of 10% of the foal's weight at day 1 and increased to 25% of the foal's weight from 10 days to weaning.

During their first week, foals should be bottlefed every 1–2 hours and then every 4–6 hours from the second week. A lamb's teat is preferred to a calf teat to allow small regular feeds. It has been shown that smaller, more frequent feeds will produce a more even growth rate. Also a smaller number of larger feeds are more likely to result in diarrhoea. Foals can also be trained to drink from a bucket.

Cleanliness is vital and used bottles should be washed and sterilised.

Foals should then begin eating solid creep feed within a few weeks and this will reduce the amount of milk required. Foals should also be fed top quality highly digestible forage.

### Creep feeding

A supplemental creep feed will ensure foals receive not only quality protein, but also essential micronutrients, especially minerals that may be lacking in pasture. If calorie intake is high from spring/summer grass then the creep feed should be a low energy/high micronutrient stud balancer. Creep feeding serves several purposes including:

- Encouraging foals to eat concentrates as early as possible
- Encouraging independence
- Helping to prevent deficiencies occurring when milk and pasture is low in certain nutrients
- Helps the foal to meet its nutritional requirements from creep feed, thereby reducing nutritional drain on the mare. This is particularly useful if she is back in foal or going to be rebred
- Helps in cases when mares are incapable of producing enough milk, which may restrict the foal's growth
- Helps in cases when the mares are excellent milkers and may push offspring into overtopped foals with growth related problems. If these foals are creep fed with a lower energy but high mineral creep feed, it is much easier to wean early if necessary.

The amount of creep feed should be followed as per the manufacturer's instructions, but a good rule of thumb is 500 g per day per month of age until six months, for foals with normal growth and bodyweight expected to mature at 500 kg plus. For heavy foals, or those with growth related problems, a lower energy creep feed is advisable.

It is important that foals are fed a creep feed formulated specifically for them and not simply allowed access to their dam's feed as this has been formulated to provide nutrients for lactation, not growth.

## Stallions

Stallions should be fed for performance in the breeding season, which will take into account the increased energy and increased (marginally) protein requirement (Figure 11.2). Performance feeds are ideal at this time with ad lib quality forage. For stallions that are good doers a forage balancer is ideal but check the vitamin E level as this can vary between products. Vitamin E and omega 3 supplements may also be beneficial. Omega 3 fatty acids are major structural elements of

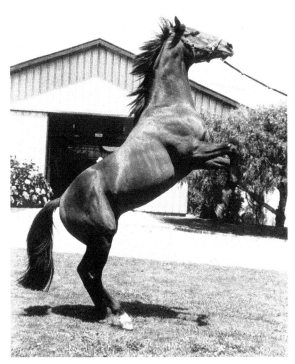

**Figure 11.2**  Stallions need plenty of energy for the breeding season. (Courtesy of Jo Prestwich)

sperm cells and therefore supplementing may help maintain stallion fertility.

## Feeding performance horses

Scientific research is providing more information with regard to feeding working horses for optimum performance. The most important aspect of feeding working horses is maintaining energy intake. Good quality forage should always be the essential basis of the feeding programme and this should be supplemented with a concentrate source supplying the appropriate fuel for the working muscles.

There are several aspects to feeding performance horses:

- Ensure optimal intake of quality forage to support the physiology of the equine digestive system and thereby maintain health and the immune system
- Meet the energy needs to match the work level and type
- Maintain an ideal bodyweight for optimum performance
- Provide optimal nutrition to aid refuelling after working or competing
- Provide all the required nutrients in the correct amounts to maintain performance and health
- Feed supplements only if required so as not to unbalance the feeding programme
- Use of supplements or injections of trace minerals/vitamins should only be undertaken with nutritional/veterinary advice.

Carbohydrates and fats are the important nutrients to provide energy for fuel for working horses. Protein is not a main source of energy. Increased protein requirements in hard working horses are generally supplied by higher intakes of concentrate feed. Dependency upon protein as a fuel source should be avoided and feed programmes for working horses should be adapted to the discipline the horses are undertaking. Feed intake must be monitored and adjusted to meet individual needs.

Several factors influence the choice of muscle fuel during work, such as availability of muscle glycogen and triglycerides (fats), fitness level of the horse, intensity and duration of work and environmental conditions.

Unfortunately total body carbohydrate stores are limited, i.e. usually substantially less than the energy required for hard work or prolonged periods of slow work. These therefore become quickly depleted during fast work and more slowly depleted during longer periods of slow speed work, leading to fatigue.

## Long distance/endurance horses

These horses primarily rely on glucose/glycogen and fatty acids from fibre and fat from the diet. They tend to be leaner types, carrying minimal excess fat, but this is not always the case.

Endurance horses and ponies should be trained to make effective use of body fat stores and adapt to using fat and fibre as feed energy sources. High levels of dietary fat help to reduce falls in blood glucose during long rides and provide slow release energy. Access to some grass at rest points is also helpful as this supplies nutrients and water. Half a litre of oil provides 18 MJ DE which is equivalent to 1.6 kg oats, however more than half a litre is difficult to achieve in practice.

Endurance horses should be fed best quality forage first and foremost, as this will increase the water and electrolytes in the hindgut. Forage should be fed little and often. Compound feeds, which are lower in starch and higher in fat and fibre, are preferred and should be fed not within 4 hours prior to a ride. High quality forage should also be offered at rest points. Electrolyte replacement is vital but overuse or incorrect use can be harmful. For example, giving a strong electrolyte solution before the horse drinks can lead to fluid being drawn into the gut to dilute the electrolytes. Electrolytes may also be given in sugar beet liquid. Horses must be trained to drink on rides to prevent dehydration.

## Show jumping/dressage

These horses need power for propulsion, consequently they are well muscled with plenty of top line. Good quality forage should provide the basis for the feeding programmes and then a medium energy performance feed should supply the rest of the energy required. If fed at less than the recommended amounts for performance, broad spectrum vitamin and mineral supplements should be added. Low starch performance feeds are preferred particularly for dressage horses to help maintain a calm temperament while working. Access to turnout and good pasture is vital to help maintain psychological health.

## Racehorses

Flat sprint horses should be fed differently from big national hunt (NH) horses. Sprinters need a supply of glucose from starch i.e. cereal based concentrates and added fat sources will probably not be very beneficial. These horses are typically more compact and square in shape with large muscle bulk. In contrast, middle distance flat racing and NH horses/point to pointers will benefit from a combination of energy sources, i.e. cereal based concentrates and a supplementary fat source. Middle distance horses usually carry some excess fat but have less muscle bulk than sprinters. Their shape is typically between the sprinter and long distance horse.

A minimum of 1% BW as top quality forage is vital for maintaining health of the digestive tract. Pre-training feeds should not be fed within 4 hours prior to work (see Eventers below). A small handful of alfalfa, hay or grass chaff can be fed for horses on early lots and their normal feed given later. Breaking yearlings need plenty of good quality forage and low starch feeds that maintain vitamin, mineral and quality amino acids to support continuing growth. Forage balancers are ideal for those carrying optimal or too much weight from the sales. For horses in light training, low starch horse and pony cubes are ideal. Once reaching mid-stage training, racehorse cubes/mix may be introduced. Racehorses need quick release energy for sprinting; it must be supplied from soluble carbohydrates but high starch concentrate feeds should be fed little and often so as not to cause hindgut acidosis. If concentrates are fed at less than the recommended amount, a broad spectrum supplement should be added. It is important that forage being fed to racehorses is analysed to make sure haylage has fermented thoroughly and to check for nutrient deficiencies. It must be of the best hygienic quality. Overfeeding supplements and injecting nutrients is a major cause of unbalanced nutrition in the racehorse. Electrolyte supplementation is vital.

## Eventers

Eventers range from novice one day to advanced three day eventers. The three day eventer should be fed top quality forage and high energy concentrate feeds. The concentrates preferred are lower starch and higher fat and fibre to provide slow release energy. Three day eventers should not be fed a high energy concentrate feed within three hours of an event as this will result in the release of insulin to store the increased blood glucose from the feed, whereas these horses need glucose to be mobilised from muscles not stored in them. High pre-exercise insulin and glucose might also limit fat oxidation and increase reliance on carbohydrates for energy. Access to forage in small but frequent amounts is also important. Electrolyte supplementation is vital and horses should be watched for signs of dehydration. After competition, horses may be fed smaller amounts of the normal concentrate feed as a warm mash to make it more appetising. Feeding some cereal starch or grain based compound feed will help muscle glycogen stores to be replenished. However, this should not be suddenly added but should be part of the every day ration in smaller amounts, which can then be increased after the cross-country. If feeding compound feeds at less than the recommended amount a performance level supplement is also required.

Novice horses and those in early training can do well on lower starch horse and pony cubes/mixes, or forage balancers moving on to performance feeds as horses get fitter.

## Feeding the older horse (veteran)

Older horses should not necessarily be swapped on to a veteran compound feed just because they reach an arbitrary age (Figure 11.3). Older horses in good condition with good dentition will be fine on the current feeding programme until signs suggest a change may be required.

Problems that may result in changes to feeding include:

- Poor dentition, tooth loss, tooth fracture, sharp teeth
- Weight loss due to inability to eat or other health reasons

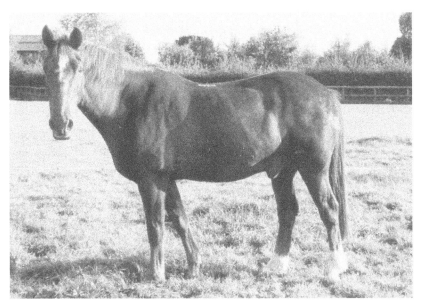

**Figure 11.3** An aged horse needs balanced nutrition to maintain health. (Courtesy L. Roberts)

- PPID (Cushing's syndrome)
- Liver dysfunction
- Kidney dysfunction
- Reduced intestinal absorption
- COPD (RAO).

Before making changes to the feed, veterinary health checks will help to assess if there are underlying disease problems that will require specific feeding. For example, liver, kidney or pituitary problems could be made worse by veteran feeds. Older horses tend to suffer from reduced absorption of nutrients. Bodyweight and condition should therefore be carefully monitored as horses can quickly lose weight.

'Healthy' veterans showing the signs of wear and tear of old age should be fed forage/concentrates 12–14% CP, lower calcium (0.6–1% as fed) and higher phosphorus (0.4–0.6% as fed). Starch and sugars should be restricted and if additional energy is required this can be supplied as vegetable oil (1 cup per day) if liver function is normal. Forage should be soft and chopped if necessary but must be digestible. Hay can be soaked for 30 minutes to soften it. Alfalfa should be avoided because of its high calcium level. Joint supplements containing glucosamine and MSM (methyl sulphonyl methane) may also be helpful as will B complex and vitamin C. However, caution is advised for horses with IR (insulin resistance) or PIPD (pituitary pars intermedia dysfunction or Cushing's syndrome) as in some trials with human patients glucosamine supplements have been shown to increase insulin resistance. Linseed oil or an omega 3 source may also be beneficial.

(For old horses with liver or kidney problems and for PIPD or IR see suggested feeding in Chapter 12.)

## Feeding overweight horses and ponies

New research indicates that overweight horses and ponies are more likely to develop insulin resistance and if allowed to remain very overweight these horses can develop Equine Metabolic Syndrome (EMS) and possibly laminitis (see Chapter 12). Horses and ponies would naturally tend to put on weight in summer and lose it in winter, but human intervention tends to prevent this natural cycle. Weight loss can be difficult to achieve in those horses that are good doers, but perseverance and exercise is the key (Figure 11.4).

Practical weight loss management is discussed at some length in Chapter 12, as are important tips for feeding laminitic horses and ponies.

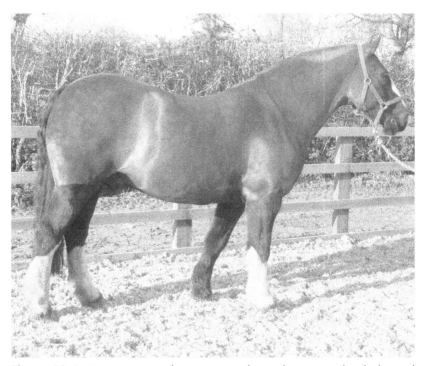

**Figure 11.4** Horses prone to being overweight can be managed with diet and exercise. (Courtesy J. Clayton)

## *Feeding for condition (underweight horse)*

If horses are in poor condition it is important to know the reason, e.g. poor management, intestinal malabsorption, worm damage or worms, ill health and/or old age. These conditions will require specific diets and veterinary or nutritional advice should be sought. It may be simply that the wrong feed or not enough is being fed. Bigger horses for example need a lot of feed. Horses that are underweight, should be checked by the vet. Horses lose body fat first and then muscle as they use protein to supply energy to maintain life processes. Horses in poor condition need a higher energy density and also quality amino acids to help build up lost muscle. Additional micronutrients such a B complex vitamins may also help as may omega 3 and prebiotic supplements such as yeast. The aim is to slowly build condition so as not to metabolically stress the horse.

Underweight horses should be fed ad lib quality forage either by pasture and/or additional hay if required. Ideally they should be fed on their own so that feed intake can be monitored. Good quality hay is preferred because it is higher in dry matter for horses with poorer appetites. A concentrate feed should be higher energy (DE at least 12 MJ/kg) and preferably these calories come more from fat and fibre as this will reduce the chance of carbohydrate overload (see hindgut acidosis in Chapter 12). Alternatively, feed a lower starch conditioning feed or performance level cube with added oil, up to 6 kg per day split between a minimum of two but preferably three feeds per day (but increase the amount slowly). This will help to reduce the GI (glycaemic index) of the feed. There are some excellent conditioning feeds now available that are lower in starch and higher in oil which also provide balanced amino acids, vitamins and minerals, so these would be preferred. Weighing the horse with a weigh tape or by the calculations given in Chapter 10 will show whether energy requirements are being exceeded, as the horse should slowly gain weight. Once the desired weight is achieved, horses should be fed a reduced energy feed. If horses are poor they shouldn't be worked (apart from light hacking) until body condition is improved. Working underweight horses hard simply uses up the energy required to improve condition.

## Feeding horses and ponies at grass

Most horses at grass will need supplementary forage in winter and a salt lick free choice. Supplementary feed may be required depending upon the quality and quantity of the grazing. Horses and ponies on poor quality grazing may need additional concentrates. A mineral block may be beneficial also but individual intake must be monitored (see Chapter 8). For good doers feeding a small amount of a low calorie forage balancer or a broad spectrum vitamin and mineral supplement in a handful of chaff daily, is ideal particularly in winter. This will make up any possible mineral deficiencies in the pasture (see Chapter 7). Additional hay/haylage should be fed in winter.

## Feeding police horses

Police horses generally have little or no access to pasture and work at a moderate level. Most police horses are good doers but exceed 16hh and need a lot of feed. Plenty of good quality forage is therefore vital. Often these horses are fed haylage but in limited amounts because the horses tend to carry too much condition. This reduces the dry matter intake as haylage contains much more water than hay, resulting in a reduced fibre intake. This can lead to colic and diarrhoea, also horses crave fibre and may begin chewing wood and licking the floors. Because of the heavy reliance upon forage for police horses, it must be nutritionally analysed. Once analysed the minimum quantity that should be fed daily can be ascertained. This can then be made up by the chosen concentrate feed. Commonly, good doers are fed reduced amounts of higher energy concentrates and so will also have reduced micronutrient intake. These horses should be fed either a forage balancer or a performance level broad spectrum vitamin and mineral supplement to make up the deficiencies. Horses requiring more energy should be fed a low starch, medium energy cube/mix, with the forage.

Electrolytes should also be fed when horses sweat. Police horses may also benefit from a prebiotic a yeast supplement and an omega 3 supplement, e.g. linseed oil.

---

**Summary points**

- All horses apart from young foals must be fed good quality forage first and foremost in the diet.
  Barren mares still need particular attention given to their diet in order to optimise chances of rebreeding.
- Pregnant mares require balanced nutrition throughout pregnancy not just in the last three months, which has been the traditional method of feeding.
- Mares fed a high fibre and oil ration balanced with important minerals vitamins and amino acids are less likely to suffer from metabolic or digestive disorders.
- A typical Thoroughbred lactating mare will produce an astonishing 11–14 kg milk per day for the first three months, these mares need highly calorific diets.
- Foals grow at extremely fast rates, particularly during the first six months of life. Daily gains of over 1 kg during the suckling phase until weaning at 6 months are very common.
- A supplemental creep feed will ensure foals receive not only quality protein, but also essential micronutrients, especially minerals that may be lacking in pasture.
- Stallions should be fed for performance in the breeding season, i.e. increased energy, vitamins and minerals.
- The most important aspect of feeding working horses is maintaining energy intake.
- Endurance horses should be trained to make effective use of body fat stores and adapt to using fat and fibre as feed energy sources.
- An absolute minimum of 1% Bodyweight given as top quality forage is vital for maintaining health of the digestive tract for performance horses.
- High starch concentrate feeds, if required, must be fed little and often so as not to cause hindgut acidosis.
- Forage should be analysed to make sure, for example, that haylage has fermented thoroughly and to check for mineral deficiencies.
- Research indicates that overweight horses and ponies are more likely to develop Insulin Resistance (IR) and if allowed to remain very overweight these horses can develop Equine Metabolic Syndrome (EMS) and possibly laminitis.

# Diet Related Problems

## LAMINITIS

Laminitis is a major cause of death in horses. This disease relates mainly to overweight horses and ponies. There are several causes of laminitis and these initially appear to be mostly unrelated to the hoof itself, these include soluble carbohydrate overload, retained placenta and trauma to the hoof such as excessive weight bearing e.g. following injury to the other forelimb. Perhaps the most common cause is pasture induced laminitis. Horses with acute laminitis have a characteristic stance, leaning backwards to take the weight off the forefeet (Figure 12.1). Laminitis is a weakening or destruction of the laminae in the hoof and in the worst case the laminae can no longer support the weight of the horse and the pedal bone rotates or sinks, even protruding through the sole of the hoof. This condition requires the urgent attention of a vet.

The key problem with the disease is that once lameness is evident, some destruction of the internal structures of the hoof has already occurred and treatment then becomes a damage limitation exercise. Prevention is therefore vital. Much research has been carried out into laminitis and its causes but perhaps the most interesting is the current work relating to equine metabolic syndrome (EMS) and insulin resistance (IR).

## Equine metabolic syndrome/insulin resistance

Equine metabolic syndrome (EMS) is actually a clinical syndrome defined by insulin resistance. There now seems to be a clear relationship between chronic obesity and insulin resistance. Although not all obese horses will develop IR, over time the risk of IR increases and, with it, associated health problems most importantly a predisposition

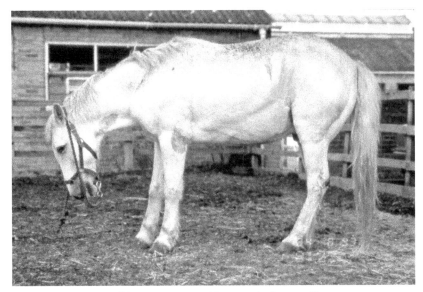

**Figure 12.1** Typical laminitic stance. (Courtesy Jo Prestwich)

to laminitis. In other words horses eventually move into EMS with IR and ultimately laminitis.

Occasionally IR can occur in horses that are lean and this condition appears much more complicated and could be related to PIDD (Cushing's syndrome) or other chronic inflammatory and therefore painful conditions.

## Insulin resistance (IR)

Insulin resistance is a reduction in the ability of the hormone insulin to stimulate body tissues. This results in an inability to effectively move glucose into the tissues from the blood thereby keeping blood glucose levels high resulting in hyperglycaemia. There appear to be two types of insulin resistance, namely:

- The pancreas secretes more insulin to compensate for the raised blood sugar to help move glucose into the tissues.
- The pancreas can no longer meet the demand for insulin and glucose levels remain high eventually causing hyperglycaemia, glucosuria (glucose in the urine) and polyuria (increased volume of urine). This is often seen in horses with PIDD (Cushing's syndrome).

The majority of horses and ponies with this problem appear to be in the first or compensated group.

EMS is an endocrine disorder, i.e. a disorder of the hormonal system of horses with chronic insulin resistance. In some cases it may develop into pituitary pars intermedia dysfunction (PPID), more commonly known as Cushing's syndrome. There is a genetic disposition to EMS and affected horses are usually very 'good doers', the type that appears to get fat on fresh air. This is probably a throwback to the times when food was scarce in winter and horses had to use up the fat stores they built up the previous summer to survive harsh winters ahead. This condition can also be seen in breeding mares showing typically cresty necks (Figure 12.2).

EMS has several characteristics:

- Insulin resistance
- Very overweight/obese
- Regional fatty areas – cresty neck and fat pads on the top of the tail and in the supraorbital fossa (dent above the eye) and swollen sheath
- Prone to laminitis
- High levels of circulating triglycerides.

If the obesity is chronic, i.e. long term, then IR becomes more likely and chronic IR increases the risk of laminitis developing.

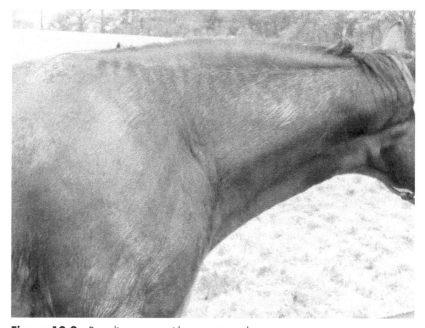

**Figure 12.2**  Breeding more with a cresty neck.

Insulin resistance has several other health implications for horses namely:

- Increased risk of laminitis (both pasture induced and toxic causes)
- Fertility problems (continuous oestrous cycle through the year no anoestrous period, longer duration of oestrous cycle)
- Increased risk of hyperlipaemia in horses and ponies in negative energy balance such as those that have gone off their feed.

It is thought that the horse's body has a limited (probably genetic) capacity to store fat. Once that limit is reached, particularly in skeletal muscle, the fat starts to interfere with insulin signalling causing IR, i.e. fat interferes with the action of insulin. This is fortunately a reversible process if caught in time, as IR can be resolved with weight loss and exercise.

In addition, from work carried out on humans it has been learnt that the overstretched fat tissue then begins to secrete substances that are pro-inflammatory into the blood. So the chronically obese horse with IR is now in a pro-inflammatory state, which makes laminitis more likely. The obese, but non-IR horse can cope with minor laminitic trigger challenges but the chronic IR horse simply can't.

It is clear that the chronically obese horse or pony is effectively on a downward spiral increasing the risk of IR, laminitis and other health problems. However, changes in management can play a large part in prevention of these problems before the situation becomes irreversible.

The aim of management is therefore to change the IR horse to an insulin sensitive state.

## Laminitis link

There are several possible mechanisms for laminitis linked to EMS and IR:

- Lack of glucose in the tissues
- Vascular dysfunction, insulin is a slow vasodilator (i.e. widens blood vessels)
- Pro-inflammatory state.

Insulin may, therefore, affect the vascular system in the hoof and ultimately affect its structural integrity. Inflammation perpetuates IR and also affects the cells in the hoof wall, by altering the natural continual remodelling system of the laminae and basement membrane, thereby effectively weakening it.

The trigger factors for starch/sugar induced laminitis are well known. However the link with IR and EMS seems very important.

Laminitis can be induced experimentally by inducing severe insulin resistance causing profound hyperinsulinaemia (high levels of blood insulin).

Pasture induced laminitis, for example, is also likely to be linked to IR.

Temperate grasses are high in water-soluble carbohydrate, which consists of differing levels of sucrose, fructose, glucose and fructans. Fructans, which consists of chains of fructose molecules joined together, is increasingly linked with laminitis. Levels of sucrose and fructans fluctuate daily in pasture, being affected by environmental factors such as intensity and duration of sunlight, temperature, water availability, soil fertility, developmental and genetic characteristics of the pasture. As with all plants, grass uses sunlight during photosynthesis to produce energy in the form of sugars. At night there is no photosynthesis (no sunlight) and the plant uses up the sugars it has made during the previous day. Sugar levels would therefore be expected to fall to their lowest levels at dawn. Fructans and sucrose exist together in a normal balance but environmental stress factors cause sucrose to be used up at a faster rate. Grass also stores fructans in the lower portion of grass plant so closely grazed pasture will be higher in fructans. If night time temperature also falls significantly, grass growth slows and more fructans accumulates.

Fructans cannot be digested in the foregut of the horse and therefore passes to the hindgut undigested and is rapidly fermented with the same consequences as discussed below.

The obese horse or pony is much more likely to consume greater amounts of pasture if allowed free access at all times. These horses often have a ravenous appetite and just don't stop eating when turned out. This can result in huge intakes of sugars at certain times of the year, which swamp the small intestine and enter the hindgut, where they are rapidly fermented leading to alteration in the microbial populations living there. This in turn increases acidity (decreases pH) leading to increased permeability of the intestinal wall. This permeability is like opening a window between the horse's circulation and the now severely unbalanced hindgut with all the endotoxins, exotoxins and vasoactive amines now able to cross this previously impermeable barrier into the horse's system, potentially triggering laminitis.

IR is involved in this scenario because researchers now think that this resultant endotoxaemia triggers a systemic inflammatory response in the horse thereby exacerbating insulin resistance. The obese horse that already has IR may have real problems handling these extra transient IR attacks caused by endotoxaemia from dietary causes and succumbs to laminitis.

Horses that are thought to be susceptible may have relatively easy veterinary tests done, including resting blood glucose and insulin levels, which will detect moderate to severe IR. This takes a ratio of glucose (mg/dl) divided by insulin (mU/l). If the number resulting is greater than 10 this is normal. If the number falls between 4.5 and 10 the horse is probably insulin resistant but compensating. If this is the case, management should be adjusted (see below) to prevent the condition deteriorating. If the result is less than 4.5 then the horse is already compromised and an immediate change in management, is required to avoid the risk of laminitis.

There is also an advanced test, which is more expensive and is a combined insulin and glucose test (CGIT). Horses with moderate to severe IR will show higher resting insulin levels. Pain is known to increase blood insulin levels and so these tests should not be done on the acutely laminitic horse as false readings may result. Some chronically obese horses and ponies may also show small degrees of pedal bone rotation on x-ray without having shown typical clinical symptoms of laminitis.

Fortunately there are management changes, which can be made to stop the escalation of obesity and IR into full-blown EMS and laminitis.

Insulin resistance can be managed by:

- Reducing sugar and other soluble carbohydrate intake.
- Reducing bodyweight in the overweight horse or pony.

To reduce IR the following management changes should be carried out:

1. Eliminate all starch based concentrates (including low-energy cool feeds) from the diet.
2. Feed later cut meadow hay with a low level of water soluble carbohydrate (WSC), i.e. sugars of less than 12%.
3. Soak hay for 30 minutes in warm water if possible before feeding to remove as many residual soluble sugars as possible.
4. Feed 2% of the horse's bodyweight as hay reducing to 1.5% if not losing weight.
5. Restrict access to pasture by strip grazing or reduce time out at grass to no longer than three to four hours. For severely affected horses and ponies, temporarily stop all access to pasture, use grass

free areas instead such as arenas until a significant reduction in bodyweight has been achieved.

6. Turning horses out for four hours per day instead of twenty four can reduce sugar intake by as much as 80%. Also try and turn out horses only at safer times of the year, i.e. not during grass flushing times, and overnight if NO frost.

7. If the horse is sound, exercise wherever possible even walking out in hand.

8. Cryotherapy is currently thought to be helpful in reducing possible damage caused by laminitis.

9. Monitor weight loss and retest for IR following weight loss programme.

10. Feed a multivitamin and mineral, performance level supplement or low starch balancer with a small amount of low calorie unmolassed chaff and unmolassed beet pulp (very dilute) if required.

11. In winter months restrict turnout on a sunny frosty morning and put horses out in the afternoon.

12. Do not feed high starch and therefore high GI coarse mixes at all and this includes some cool mixes (see Chapter 7).

These management tools may also be applied to overweight laminitics or those predisposed to the disease to help reduce further incidents. For underweight laminitics, energy should be supplied as fat and fibre or low starch horse and pony cubes/fibre based compounds (not cool mixes which may be high starch). Supplementation with a high performance vitamin and mineral supplement may be useful while horses are in the painful acute stages of the disease.

Managing lean horses with IR is more problematical. Calories must be provided via fat (oil) and digestible fibre, i.e. low starch and sugars as above, limited grass and low WSC hay. Feeds should be made up of unmolassed beet pulp, low sugar chaff, vegetable or linseed oil and a good vitamin and mineral supplement or low starch balancer.

# PPID OR CUSHING'S

Pituitary pars intermedia dysfunction (PPID) or Cushing's syndrome as it used to be known is very common in older horses and ponies over 15 years of age. PPID refers to abnormal function of a distinct area of the pituitary gland known as the pars intermedia lobe. This is quite complicated as the pituitary gland is responsible for secreting many activating hormones into the blood, they then affect other organ/s or system/s elsewhere such as the adrenal gland. Horses with PPID have an enlarged pituitary gland.

The normal pituitary gland has three lobes each producing different hormones for the horse's body. The normal pars intermedia produces hormones under instruction from the hypothalamus that sits above it at the base of the brain. Hormones produced from the pars intermedia affect skin colour, appetite, fat metabolism and can stimulate insulin release. Adrenocorticotrophic hormone (ACTH), for example, causes the adrenal gland near the kidney to produce the steroid hormone cortisol. If ACTH production by the pituitary gland is abnormal, it can hyperstimulate the adrenal gland and this is known as hyperadreno-corticism. Continual overproduction of cortisol then affects many parts of the horse's body such as hair coat, feet, etc. When the pars interme-dia is not functioning properly hormone production becomes abnor-mal. Hormone dysregulation therefore may cause several metabolic type problems including fat storage problems and insulin resistance (see above). Increasing activity of these hormones secreted from the abnormal pars intermedia results in increased symptoms in autumn, for example, when Cushing's laminitis may be more common. Other signs of PPID include:

- Excessive thirst and urination
- Long curly winter coat that is not shed in summer
- Muscle wasting
- Pot bellied appearance
- Recurrent infections of the sole of the hoof, respiratory tract and skin
- Lethargy.

Diagnosis of Cushing's is undertaken through veterinary tests for spe-cific hormones and from a history of symptoms.

## EXERTIONAL RHABDOMYOLYSIS

Exertional rhabdomyolysis (ER) is a common problem for working horses. In the past this painful muscular condition was referred to by many names including tying-up, set fast, azoturia and monday morning disease – all of which have a common theme, i.e. muscle pain and cramps of varying degrees.

Exertional rhabdomyolysis in horses refers specifically to muscle pain associated with exercise. It may be sporadic, meaning that horses have occasional episodes, or chronic i.e. repeated episodes, which may put the working career of the horse in jeopardy. Recent work now refers to two types of repeated episodes of ER:

- PSSM – polysaccharide storage myopathy – affects mainly quarter horses, warmbloods, draft breeds
- Recurrent ER – affects thoroughbreds (TBs) in training, Arabs and standardbreds.

PSSM refers to abnormal metabolism of glycogen within the muscle, whereas in other horses recurrent ER has been linked to abnormal calcium regulation within the muscle cells or contractile problems within the muscle fibres.

Horses suffering from PSSM have problems storing and utilising glucose and its storage form glycogen. In practice though, in cases of both PSSM and recurrent ER, a reduction in starch/sugar levels within feed and possibly increased oil are helpful in managing the problem. In working horses, there are also other important dietary/management factors which may be causing or contributing to the problem.

The disease process results in breakdown of muscle cells causing massive inflammation and pain. Because muscle cells break down, their contents are released into the blood hence the increases seen in plasma creatine kinase (CK) and aspartate aminotransferase or aspartate trans-aminase (AST). Blood tests give information regarding the severity of the problem. In particularly severe cases the urine can turn a dark brown colour as the kidneys excrete myoglobin released from the break-down of muscle cells and this may further cause kidney damage.

Rhabdomyolysis may occur when a horse is exercised after a rest day (known as set fast, azoturia or monday morning disease) typically when hard feed (usually high in cereal starch) has not been reduced and/or the horse has been stabled on the rest day without any exercise.

The onset of ER is linked to factors such as sex, age, temperament, exercise levels and also lameness. Exertional rhabdomyolysis usually occurs soon after exercise. The typical signs include initial stiffness of the muscles, followed by sweating; lameness behind and the muscles of the hindquarters feel hard and painful to the touch. This may then develop further to the horse not being able to move, being in severe pain and with an increased breathing rate. In some competition horses, a subclinical problem may occur with horses simply showing poor tolerance to training, reduced stamina and horses not being able to finish competitions.

Blood tests show raised CK and AST levels, with increased values corresponding to high levels of muscle damage. If AST levels remain higher than normal over time, this could be as a result of previous episodes. In severe cases of recurrent exertional rhabdomyolysis (RER), there may be electrolyte irregularities such as low sodium, calcium and chloride levels or high levels of potassium and phosphorus. These may result from excessive sweating or movement of electrolytes from damaged muscle cells, resulting in metabolic alkalosis as the horse's body tries to compensate for the high blood chloride levels.

Horses on high cereal starch feeds such as coarse mixes but also some cubes are also more likely to suffer, as are horses with low grade lameness.

Abnormal calcium regulation within the muscle cells taking place intermittently during exercise is also a cause. In addition abnormal sensitivity to potassium has been found in horses with the problem. High intakes of forage combined with excessive electrolyte supplements may lead to excessively high potassium intakes, (not usually a problem for racehorses in training).

Management of horses with RER can help to reduce the incidence. In practice, reducing excitement for nervous types is known to help, as does daily turnout. The use of horse walkers depends upon the individual horse as some continue to suffer from ER while on the walker. Rest days should be avoided for blood tests show that CK levels increase for horses exercised after a day of rest. Horses should be turned out on rest days, with a good rug if necessary. It is essential that horses warm up before exercise and are allowed to gradually cool down afterwards.

Injecting or supplementing with vitamin E and/or selenium has not been shown to help ER. However, other dietary changes such as feeding lower cereal starch feeds and the addition of oil to each feed seems to reduce the glycaemic response. High energy haylage (cut early in the season) should also be avoided and if possible hay fed instead. Ensuring adequate salt intake by providing free choice salt licks/blocks and electrolytes when horses freely sweat after exercise is important. Feeding an electrolyte containing calcium gluconate could be helpful as this calcium source is highly available. As lactic acidosis is not a cause of this disease the feeding of sodium bicarbonate and dimethyglycine does not appear to be necessary.

## FEED ALLERGIES

Allergic reactions in horses are particularly common. These reactions can make horses quite subdued. Many horses have episodic allergic reactions but occasionally some horses will develop regular recur-

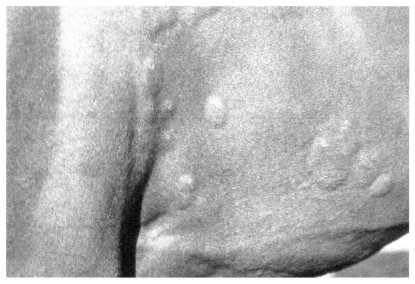

**Figure 12.3** Urticarial hives; soft swellings under the skin. This figure was published in *Diseases and Disorders of the Horse*, Knottenbelt and Pascoe. Copyright: Elsevier (1994).

rences of the condition. Symptoms of feed allergies are extremely inconsistent, varying from the soft typical urticarial type swellings (hives) just under the skin (Figure 12.3) to small hard bumps or papules. The swellings or lumps may be very itchy (pruritis) or not itchy at all. When horses are really itchy they may rub themselves raw. Alopecia may also follow resulting in significant hair loss. Fluid from these soft lumps may eventually drain downwards underneath the skin resulting in large fluid filled areas between the front legs or under the belly. Allergies may be localised or cover the whole body or significant parts of it. Most horses suffering from allergies do not develop a temperature, but it is important to note that occasionally some viral infections may result in lumps appearing.

Allergic reactions or hypersensitivities are a result of the horse becoming sensitised to at least one antigen. Recent research suggests that substances known as glycoproteins present in many fresh and prepared feeds and supplements may act as a base for these antigens. However, researchers do not know which part of the glycoprotein or even which glycoprotein is causing the problem. Allergic hives are often called protein bumps, but it is not the amount of protein causing the problem, rather it is a single glycoprotein or allergen that causes the hypersensitivity. These proteins are often found within cereals particularly barley or wheat. Following a suspected feed causing allergic reaction in the horse, a full history should be taken of every-thing the horse has eaten and note whether there have been any recent changes to the diet. Check also if the horse has been recently vaccinated or wormed or the forage source changed or if the horse is being treated with pharmaceutical drugs. Horses with repeated allergic reactions may benefit from intradermal allergen testing although this has vari-able results with false positives and negatives. Horses with recurrent feed allergy problems should be placed on an elimination diet to try and determine the source of the problem. The elimination diet involves removing cereals from the ration. Start with forage alone consisting of grass hay or alfalfa to appetite within reason. If these are a problem a non-straw hay replacer may be used. A limestone based performance level vitamin and mineral supplement can also be fed to maintain micronutrient intake. Many supplements and additives use cereal-based carriers so the manufacturer should be contacted for more infor-mation. Grass pellets are a good choice being a single ingredient pellet. If the horse is allergic to a feed ingredient this diet should result in improvement of symptoms within four weeks. Following this a single ingredient from the horse's previous ration may be reintroduced every week. If and when identified, the problem ingredient can be avoided. However, horses may be allergic to more than one allergen.

Antihistamines and glucocorticoid therapy are not useful long term and the elimination diet is probably the best route even though it is time consuming.

## GASTRIC ULCERS OR EGUS

Gastric ulcers are extremely common in performance horses, particu-larly those in training, however it is now thought they are common in other horses including broodmares and foals. In broodmares, this may be related to high intakes of compound feeds.

Ulcers at the very least may result in ill health and at worst result in death. A horse can develop gastric ulcers in as little as three days.

Gastric ulcers, or to give the technical name, equine gastric ulcer syndrome (EGUS), are a serious health problem in both adult horses and foals. It is suggested that as many as 80–90% of horses in training may have gastric lesions at any one time.

Ulceration may be so severe as to cause perforation, resulting in release of stomach contents into the abdomen usually causing perito-nitis and possible loss of the horse. EGUS actually refers to injury to the horse's stomach lining caused mainly by acid secretion or more general changes to the natural protection of the lining of the stomach (mucosa). Horses removed from the constant foraging of natural fibre type feeds, seem to be at the highest risk of developing EGUS.

## Causes

EGUS is a multifactorial problem. Traditional feeding practices of minimal forage and high grain rations are a major factor. Recently it is thought that volatile fatty acids (VFAs) produced by microbial fermentation of soluble carbohydrates such as cereal starch may be contributing to damage of the gastric lining causing ulcers. Both large amounts of cereal based feeds and periods of fasting result in elevated levels of stomach acid. Horses eating forage based diets chew far more and produce greater amounts of saliva. This saliva helps to naturally buffer or neutralise the acid in the stomach. Alfalfa has been shown to help reduce severity and incidence of gastric ulcers although it is not a treatment. Cereal feeds also may increase production of the hormone gastrin, which stimulates the release of gastric acid further.

Some medications such as NSAIDs (non-steroidal anti-inflammatory drugs), which include phenylbutazone and flunixine meglumine, may, if given in excess, cause EGUS. The effect of these drugs seems to be more common in the lower stomach area known as the pyloric region. However, at recommended dosage rates this is unlikely to result in problems in adult horses, but in foals less than one year of age these drugs may result in ulcers.

## Symptoms of EGUS

The damage to the stomach lining caused by acid in the stomach may result in mild to great discomfort and consequent reduced performance. Definite diagnosis requires endoscopy by the veterinary surgeon.

### Foals

- Intermittent nursing
- Intermittent colic
- Pot belly appearance
- Lying on back
- Diarrhoea
- Excess salivation
- Teeth grinding.

*Adult horses*

- Reduced appetite, failure to finish grain feed
- Weight loss
- Decreased performance
- Dull rough coat
- Lethargy, depression
- Low grade, but frequent colic symptoms
- Teeth grinding.

Treatment involves a range of approaches including drug therapy and management changes. It is well known that horses at pasture in general do not suffer from ulcers. Ulcers will normally heal when horses are turned out to pasture, if they are not too severe.

The main drug treatments are aimed at inhibiting acid secretion – e.g. Gastrogard (omeprazole paste) and Zantac (ranitidine). Treatments can be expensive, particularly if used for long-term treatment and omeprazole is expensive. The presence of a high fibre food in the stomach may help to neutralise stomach acid. High fibre foods will also encourage chewing and the production of increased amounts of acid buffering saliva. Researchers in Tennessee have shown that alfalfa may actually have a more protective effect than other forages because of its high protein and calcium content giving improved buffering properties.

There has been some research into the use of electrolyte pastes for endurance and eventing horses both prior to and during competitions. Researchers now think that thess may exacerbate gastric ulcers. Adding a cup of corn oil to a grain feed is also thought to reduce the amount of acid produced by the stomach and this could be a good management tool.

## CHOKE/OESOPHAGEAL OBSTRUCTION

Choke is caused by horses swallowing (often bolting) food that is too dry or coarse, such as coarse dry hay/straw. Some food may swell rapidly once swallowed and mixed with saliva and this may cause choke. Horses with injuries or that have been sedated may also have problems with choke. Horses that are choking can still breathe (unlike humans with choke). The signs include drooling or feed material coming from the nostrils and mouth. In severe cases the oesophagus may rupture although this is rare.

Horses require veterinary attention whereby a tube is passed down to try and ease the blockage into the stomach. An injection may be given to relax the muscles of the oesophagus. A possible complication is pneumonia if some of the blocked food becomes aspirated on to the lungs. Following choke, feeds should be fed wet for a while or horses should be just allowed to graze. The teeth and mouth should be checked and attention given if required. Also avoid very fibrous feeds such as straw or very late cut hay and soak cubes before feeding.

# HINDGUT ACIDOSIS

Feeding high levels of cereal starch feeds or pastures rich in fructans can result in subclinical hindgut acidosis. This can make horses feel unwell and lose appetite. It may also result in mild colic symptoms, and weight loss with a general poor performance syndrome.

Subclinical acidosis is thought to follow ingestion of large cereal starch containing compound feed or pastures rich in fructans. This high volume of starch overwhelms the stomach and small intestine, which cannot therefore digest it all, leading to undigested starch entering the hindgut where it is rapidly fermented. Fructans bypasses the foregut, as the horse does not have enzymes to digest it and thereby passes into the hindgut where it is rapidly fermented. The products of this rapid fermentation are Volatile Fatty Acids (VFAs) and lactic acid which cause a significant rise in caecum and colon acidity, i.e. a fall in pH. Lactic acid is much stronger than VFAs and so is more likely to cause damage to the mucosa of the caecum and colon, resulting in inflammation, discomfort and decreased appetite.

The drop in pH also creates an unfavourable environment for the many beneficial microbes (e.g. cellulolytic bacteria) that are required for digestion of fibre. These require a pH of around 6.5–7.0 for optimal fibre digestion. As the pH falls below 6.0 the bacteria cannot function and begin to die off, producing substantial changes in the hindgut environment, i.e. dysbiosis. In the long term, the prolonged exposure of the lining of the gut to increased acidity will cause damage but may also affect absorption of important nutrients through the intestinal wall. More severe falls in pH may lead to death of huge numbers of bacteria, which release endotoxins possibly causing laminitis. Recent research suggests that hindgut acidosis may increase the incidence of certain stereotypical behaviours such as box walking, weaving, cribbing and chewing wood.

A stable hindgut microbial environment is required for optimal feed efficiency. Horses with inefficient digestive systems will also tend to lose weight and condition and are typically known as 'poor doers'. The solution that can help to reduce the incidence of dysbiosis and subclinical acidosis is to limit the amount of starch fed per meal and also add a protected buffer that reaches the hindgut and helps to prevent the fall in pH.

## COLIC

This is one of the most common veterinary problems in horses and can be fatal. Colic describes abdominal pain and there are a huge variety of causes, which can make veterinary diagnosis challenging. Epidemiological studies have shown that feeding mismanagement increases the colic risk significantly, such as:

• Lack of water
• Poor dentition
• Over-consumption of high starch feed causing acidosis
• Changes in forage, e.g. pasture to hay/haylage.

Horses with colic often roll excessively to help relieve the pain (Figure 12.4). Parasites such as large and small strongyles and tapeworm can

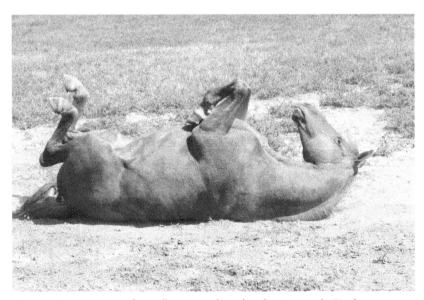

**Figure 12.4**   Horses often roll excessively with colic. Copyright Fotolia.

also cause colic. Encysted small strongyle larvae may embed in the intestinal wall.

Colic pain is usually derived from distension of the stomach or intestinal walls caused by accumulation of gas and/or fluid or food or by a blockage or cessation of normal gut movement. Approximately 90% of colics react well to medical treatment but 10% will require surgery. This 10% will have a better prognosis if the cause is found early and surgery is consequently performed quickly.

Horses with colic can exhibit extreme pain and veterinary intervention is essential to prevent the situation deteriorating.

Symptoms of colic include:

- Anorexia, lack of appetite
- Few or no droppings
- Lethargy
- Looking at flanks
- Pawing ground
- Kicking belly
- Rolling excessively
- Patchy sweating
- Increased respiratory rate
- Increased heart rate.

The source of colic is within the digestive tract from the stomach onward and types of colic include:

- Spasmodic colic
- Parasitic causes
- Stomach – motility loss leading to gas production from fermentation soon after feeding
- Small intestine – e.g. ileal impaction, strangulated pedunculated lipoma, enteritis in small intestine, grass sickness, hernia
- Large Intestine – e.g. impaction at the pelvic flexure, right dorsal or left dorsal colon displacement, sand impaction, torsion of large intestine also known as volvulus and gas or tympanic colic.

The small intestine secretes large volumes of liquid every day to help the digestive process. Obstruction of the small intestine therefore rapidly leads to build-up of secreted fluid and distension and pain. In the small intestine the ileum appears predisposed to impaction problems as food passes through the ileocaecal valve into the caecum. However, in the large intestine, the transit time is slow to allow time for thorough microbial fermentation of fibre. Large volumes of gas are produced during this fermentation so obstruction of the large intestine rapidly results in gas build-up and therefore distension and pain. Digesta in the large intestine tends to be drier than in the small intestine as water is absorbed and so impactions of very coarse fibrous food are more common.

Spasmodic colic is probably the most common cause of colic, it tends to be mild and short in duration, often no longer than a couple of hours. Signs of pain are more of discomfort rather than severe. Medical treatment of pain killing injections usually results in fairly swift resolution. Loud rumbling sounds in the gut are associated with spasmodic colic. Spasmodic colic can also be caused by parasites, in particular tapeworm, and changes in feed including forage.

## Tympanic colic

This is commonly due to overproduction of gas in the large intestine and common causes include sudden changes in diet, lush pasture, or overfeeding of high starch concentrates.

## Impaction of pelvic flexure

The most commonly diagnosed colic in the large intestine, this can be felt by rectal palpation and once diagnosed, can be effectively treated with lubricants and medical treatment. The pelvic flexure is a point at which there is a sudden change in direction and a narrowing of the large intestine at the same point and food can become impacted at this point. This often occurs with dietary changes such as pasture to fibrous stermmy woody hay or haylage.

## Sand colic

Sand accumulates in the large intestine and this is more common in the USA and dry sandy areas. Horses fed hay on sand arenas, for example, can take in too much sand. Sand has to be removed through surgery but the prognosis is good.

## Torsion or volvulus of the large intestine

This is often seen in mares following birth and in horses with a recent change in diet. The large intestine twists on itself causing strangulation, cutting off the blood supply and therefore causing death of intestinal tissue. This is a veterinary emergency and horses quickly go into endotoxaemic shock. Horses may die within a few hours if not treated. Prognosis is often guarded.

## Feeding horses post-colic

If colic surgery has taken place without resection (removal of a portion of the gut), then good quality forage should be introduced little and often as soon as the horse can eat, this will help stimulate the gut to move. When the horse is able to eat voluntarily following surgery, a maintenance ration high in quality fibre and water content should follow with additional vitamins and minerals for a week or so. Many vets advocate not feeding any cereal feeds at this time, as this will help hindgut function to return to normal. Cereal concentrates can be introduced from two weeks, but in small amounts. If resection has been carried out, special dietary requirements will be necessary depending upon which part of the gut has been resected. In general, horses will have an increased need for B vitamins, phosphorus and quality amino acids and a reduced capacity for fibre digestion.

If the small intestine is resected, emphasis on the large intestine will be needed. The amount of cereals should be reduced, as the small intestine is the primary site for simple carbohydrate digestion. Feed alfalfa and beet pulp and oil (if the ileum is fully intact); If the ileum has been resected horses will also need injectable vitamins A and E and possibly K and extra calcium as this is a major site of calcium absorption.

Following colic not requiring surgery, once the colic has stopped (during which water and feed is usually withheld) normal feed can be reintroduced at a low level, building up to pre-colic intakes unless the current feed regime has caused the colic in the first place! This might be the case where large amounts of cereal concentrates are fed.

## GRASS SICKNESS

This disease affects horses, ponies and donkeys. It causes gut paralysis and can be fatal. The disease occurs almost exclusively in horses at grass.

Grass sickness has three forms, acute, subacute and chronic, with a considerable overlap of symptoms. In acute grass sickness the symptoms are severe and horses often die or are euthanased within a couple of days.

Severe gut paralysis leads to signs of colic including rolling, pawing at the ground and looking at the flanks, difficulty in swallowing and drooling of saliva.

Foul smelling fluid may appear at the nostrils and severe constipation also occurs. In subacute grass sickness horses have difficulty swallowing, mild colic, sweating and muscle tremors. These horses may die within seven days. In the chronic form of the disease the symptoms are more insidious in onset: lack of appetite, weight loss and emaciation. Some chronic cases are treatable depending upon the symptoms but horses take a long time to recover.

Grass sickness has been a problem for many years. Increasing evidence points to *Clostridium botulinum* type C as the cause. This is different from the bacterium that causes botulism, namely type B. Under certain environmental conditions the bacterium can produce a range of toxins, which destroy nerve cells in the horse's intestine, drastically reducing intestinal function. Acute grass sickness is often fatal. Most cases of grass sickness occur in April/May with another peak in September/October. It is well known that certain premises, or even fields within single premises, are associated with the occurrence of grass sickness cases. Horses which have recently moved to previously affected premises are more likely to develop the disease in the first couple of months. Commonly, only one horse is affected at a time but 'outbreaks' of the disease with several cases in a period of a few weeks may occur.

## FEEDING SICK/INJURED HORSES

Severe trauma such as burns, serious accidents and acute infections will drastically increase the need for energy, quality amino acids and vitamins whereas nutrient needs for common respiratory viruses or less serious injuries will be fewer. Vitamin C (10 g/day) is a particularly useful supplement for these horses to help maintain the immune system during the injury or illness. Maintaining intake of important antioxidants including vitamin E and selenium is also essential. It is important to maintain intake of nutrients to aid healing and uphold immune function.

Maintaining quality forage intake will help provide calories and keep the digestive tract working normally for horses on box rest. Feeding cool mixes or cubes is common practice, but they often contain high starch levels, which may result in muscular problems. The starch content should be less than 10% in the chosen feed.

Horses that are in pain may quickly lose their appetite at a time when nutrition is vital. Pain and/or a high temperature will often prevent horses eating and unfortunately this soon leads to horses breaking down their own body tissues to produce energy, a process known as catabolism. This process may kick in from as little as 24 hours without food. Catabolism soon produces further problems including weakness, muscle wastage, (including heart muscle) reduced repair and healing and suppression of the immune system. Horses with a poor appetite may also benefit from supplementation with B complex vitamins, as will horses that have been treated with antibiotics.

For horses that cannot eat, for example post-operative or severely sick horses, these animals will need to be fed in the short term either via a nasogastric tube as required or given parenteral nutrition intra-venously. This requires veterinary supervision and as soon as physi-cally possible, horses should then be given feed orally to maintain health of the digestive tract.

Horses in acute or chronic pain may benefit from a short period of pain relief (analgesia) and this should again be discussed with the vet.

Horses should be offered little and often to tempt them to eat. For horses that can be walked out in hand, access to grazing is an appetite stimulant; otherwise small amounts of fresh grass can be picked and offered straight away. The addition of one or more of apple juice, carrot juice, molassed beet pulp, alfalfa, chopped apples and carrots may help to stimulate the horse to eat and the addition of warm water will help release the aromas to try and tempt the horse to eat.

## LIVER (HEPATIC) DISEASE

The liver has many important functions including glucose synthesis from fat and protein and detoxification. Chronic liver disease tends to result in weight loss caused by loss of appetite. Low plasma sugar and insulin resistance are common. Feeding horses with liver disease is aimed at reducing the liver's workload, in particular reducing ammonia build-up by feeding a low protein ration. This includes supplementing with fat soluble vitamins A, D, E and K and short branch chain amino acids (BCAAs) such as valine, leucine and isoleucine. Aromatic amino acids should be low. Sugar beet, wheat bran, linseed and maize all contain good levels of BCAAs. The diet should be low protein 8–10% but contain higher levels of high GI (glycaemic Index) feeds such as cereals (fed little and often). Alfalfa should be avoided because of its high protein content. Additional B complex vitamins and vitamin C are also helpful as the damage liver is not able to make enough vitamin C. Alfalfa and soya are too high in protein.

## KIDNEY (RENAL) DISEASE

Kidneys are vital for water and electrolyte balance and removing nitrogenous waste from the body. Acute renal failure results in azotaemia (nitrogenous substances in the plasma) and disruption to electrolyte and fluid balance. Chronic kidney problems are sometimes seen in veteran horses causing anorexia, weight loss and lethargy. The kidneys are also vital for removing excess calcium from the body and so chronic kidney problems can result in increases in blood calcium.

Horses with renal disease should be fed in a similar way to those with liver disease, i.e. low protein diet (<10% CP). A positive energy balance should be maintained to prevent protein breakdown as a source of energy. As kidneys are the primary sites of calcium excretion, feeds rich in calcium such as alfalfa and beet pulp may result in the accumulation of calcium crystals in the kidneys, which may form kidney stones. Wheat bran and rice bran should be avoided. Feed quality meadow hay and supplemented cereals little and often. Feed supplementary B complex vitamins especially thiamine (B1). Free choice salt should also be made available.

## DIARRHOEA

In adult horses diarrhoea is usually a result of large bowel disease. It often follows sudden changes in diet such as a change in forage or hard feed although this is often temporary. Turnout on spring grass often brings loose droppings – again usually temporary. The loose droppings are not the result of the high water content of grass as frequently thought but are due to high sugars including fructans and low fibre.

The high soluble carbohydrate intake results in hindgut acidosis, causing water to be secreted into the hindgut from the body thereby increasing water content of the droppings. Changes to the hindgut microbes may also result in toxins being produced, which irritate the gut lining causing more mucus to be produced.

If diarrhoea continues for more than a couple of days horses should be supplemented with B vitamins and electrolytes. Feeding ad lib hay, salt and water is recommended if the diarrhoea follows treatment with antibiotics. High GI feeds such as starchy cereal mixes (even cool mixes) should be avoided. Preprobiotics may also be beneficial. A vet should investigate foals suffering from acute diarrhoea, as serious illness and even death can quickly result from severe dehydration.

# LYMPHANGITIS

The lymphatic system is a major part of the immune system. Lymph is a watery fluid that leaks out of blood vessels into spaces between body tissues and then is returned by a series of lymph vessels before being returned to the blood. Lymph is circulated not by the heart but by muscle movement or massage. Excessive feeding combined with too little exercise leads to swelling, particularly of the lower hindlimbs where lymph fluid accumulates. This is because the muscle massage cannot return the excessive lymph, as the horse is not moving about. This also often follows viral infections or damage to blood capillaries and lymph vessels by toxins following bacterial infections causing them to become excessively leaky. Lymphangitis often follows mud fever that has breached the skin barrier. Treatment involves changing the diet if too excessive or treating the bacterial/viral infection or mud fever if possible. Horses should be walked out in hand if it is not possible to turn them out.

# DEVELOPMENTAL ORTHOPAEDIC DISEASE

Developmental orthopaedic disease (DOD) is a term given to encompass all general growth disturbances to the horse's skeletal system, which include dyschondroplasia (DCP), osteochondrosis (OC) and osteochondritis dissecans (OCD). Physitis (otherwise known as epiphysitis or physeal dysplasia), angular limb deformities (flexural deformities and contracted tendons), and wobbler syndrome are included under the DOD name. DOD is sometimes referred to as developmental skeletal problems (DSP).

Dyschondroplasia is a general term for the disturbance of the maturation process of cartilage to bone in young horses. Common early visible signs include 'lumpy' joints, particularly the fetlocks and knees. The lumps begin to appear above and/or below the joints and affect both sides or just one side. Sometimes these lumpy joints are accompanied by heat and/or lameness. If severe the whole joint can appear round like a tennis ball. Angular limb deformities and contracted tendons are also visible signs of problems (Figure 12.5) but OC and OCD may often

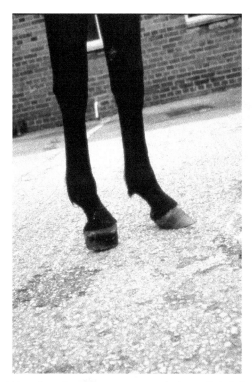

**Figure 12.5** Weanling showing a contracted deep digital flexor tendon. This figure was published in *Diseases and Disorders of the Horse*, Knottenbelt and Pascoe. Copyright: Elsevier (1994).

lie latent until the problem is so progressed that external clinical symptoms such as lameness and swelling appear. The earlier these problems are recognised and steps taken to identify possible causes, then the greater the chance of correction. Recent research has implicated high cereal starch rations as being a possible cause of DOD. This is thought to be related to the hormone insulin, which when released in high concentrations following a relatively large cereal (starch) feed may further affect growth hormone. Feeding high protein feeds does not cause DOD, but overfeeding high energy feeds may do so.

Low starch, specially formulated nutritionally balanced feeds are essential for foals as trace mineral deficiencies in pasture are common. Research indicates that both copper and zinc deficiencies also play vital roles in DOD. Supplementing new born foals with excess copper appears not as effective as ensuring copper levels are optimum for the pregnant mare (and therefore foetus) throughout gestation, i.e. from conception to foaling and through lactation.

The zinc to copper ratio is also important as high levels of zinc and marginal copper levels can result in DOD.

New areas of research involving the role of high carbohydrate (e.g. cereal\starch) feeding of young foals and high blood sugar and insulin levels may throw more light on the causes of DOD.

## POOR HOOF HORN QUALITY

Some horses and ponies seem to be particularly prone to poor hoof quality. Figure 12.6 shows a badly cracked hoof.

Currently, there are many supplements on the market aimed at improving hoof horn quality, often with little research behind them. Hoof horn grows continuously from the coronet band and this growth requires many different nutrients, including calcium, zinc, manganese, selenium, copper, vitamin A, vitamin E and perhaps the most widely known, biotin.

Certainly, any ration that is deficient in one of more of these essential nutrients will affect the quality of the new hoof horn laid down. Horses that are malnourished tend to have poor hooves and a poor coat due to the overall effect of deficiencies within the body. Once given a bal-

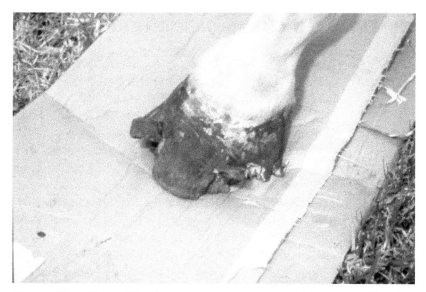

**Figure 12.6** Cracked hoof in very poor condition. This figure was published in *Diseases and Disorders of the Horse*, Knottenbelt and Pascoe. Copyright: Elsevier (1994).

anced ration these horses often start to show improvement in the hoof horn quality. Horses out on good pasture are unlikely to be low in biotin and therefore this is probably not the primary cause of poor feet. However, low zinc and/or copper may be a problem and pasture levels should be checked. The structural protein of skin is keratin and so it is for hoof horn. There are other complex proteins associated with hoof horn. Sulphur containing amino acids such as methionine, cysteine and cystine are needed for cross-linking in larger proteins such as keratin. A deficiency in one or more of these amino acids and lysine will lead to poor growth and problems with poor hoof and skin condition.

Stabled horses on low forage rations such as competition horses may be short of biotin, given that the stress of working may reduce manufacture of B vitamins within the large intestine. If horses are fed high levels of a nutritionally balanced feed, biotin should be supplied in sufficient quantities by the feed. For horses with poor hoof horn, clean bedding at all times is a must and these horses may benefit from supplementation with 20 mg daily of biotin for at least nine months. Other important nutrients may be lacking as discussed previously, but too little calcium may be a factor in horses fed oats/bran/cereal based diets that have not been adequately balanced.

## CRIBBING (CRIB BITING), WIND SUCKING, WOOD CHEWING, TAIL CHEWING, SOIL LICKING

These are known as stereotypies and include crib biting and wind sucking, although wood chewing is not a stereotypy it may lead to crib biting and wind sucking.

Recent research suggests that hindgut acidosis may increase the incidence of these stereotypical behaviours, (see p. 199).

Crib biting occurs when horses grasp a fixed object such as the stable door or fence post with their incisors pulling back and sucking air into the windpipe and grunting. This causes excessive wear to the incisors or front teeth. Wind sucking is the same but the horse does not grasp anything. Surgery can now be carried out to stop horses cribbing or wind sucking although this is in its infancy.

Research has shown that foals that begin to crib bite spend more time trying to suckle their dams and this may be because the milk is in short supply and/or the foal is hungry. Lack of milk and production of acid in the stomach may also result in gastric ulcers. Low starch creep feeds are therefore preferred for foals. Horses that crib or wind suck should

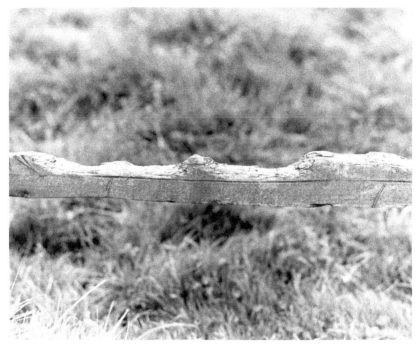

**Figure 12.7**   Well chewed fence due to fibre or mineral deficiency.

have access to quality fibre at all times and be fed low starch concentrate feeds.

Wood chewing is often due to lack of fibre or salt. Some wood for fencing is salt treated and may encourage chewing (Figure 12.7). If horses are chewing the fencing when out at pasture, salt should be provided and also hay especially in spring when fibre levels are low. Tail chewing is often the result of salt or another mineral deficiency, and the overall ration should be checked.

Licking the soil or geophagia is possibly a sign of mineral deficiency, particularly salt.

---

**Summary points**

- Insulin resistance is a reduction in the ability of the hormone insulin to stimulate body tissues.
- Prevention of laminitis is preferred to treatment.
- Cryotherapy is a new prevention/treatment for laminitis.
- The obese horse or pony is much more likely to consume greater amounts of pasture, if allowed free access at all times.
- Exertional rhabdomyolysis (ER) in horses refers specifically to muscle pain associated with exercise.
- Allergic reactions in horses are fairly common, making horses quite subdued.
- Gastric ulcers are a serious health problem in both adult horses and foals.
- Horses with renal disease should be fed in a similar way to those with liver disease, i.e. low protein diet (<10% CP).
- Horses that are choking can still breathe (unlike humans with choke).
- Feeding high levels of cereal starch feeds or pastures rich in fructans can result in subclinical hindgut acidosis.
- DOD is not caused by feeding too much protein, but too much cereal starch may increase the incidence of DOD.
- Colic is one of the most common veterinary problems in horses and can be fatal.
- Feeding mismanagement increases the colic risk significantly.
- Grass sickness has been a problem for many years. Increasing evidence points to *Clostridium botulinum* type C as the cause.
- Recent research suggests that hindgut acidosis may increase the incidence of crib biting and wind sucking.

# Appendix 1
# Nutritional Requirements Tables

All data in the tables of this appendix are reprinted with permission from the National Academies Press, Copyright 2007, National Academy of Sciences.

# DAILY NUTRIENT REQUIREMENTS OF PONIES WEIGHING 200KG OR THOSE EXPECTED TO MATURE AT THIS WEIGHT

(Major nutrients from NRC Nutrient Requirements of Horses 2007)

| | Weight kg | DE Mcal | DE MJ | CP g | Lysine g | Ca g | P g | Mg g | K g | Na g | Cu mg | Se mg | Zn mg | Vit A IU | Vit D IU | Vit E IU |
|---|---|---|---|---|---|---|---|---|---|---|---|---|---|---|---|---|
| Adult maintenance average | 200 | 6.7 | 28.1 | 252 | 10.8 | 8.0 | 5.6 | 3.0 | 10.0 | 4.0 | 40.0 | 0.4 | 160.0 | 6,000 | 1320 | 200 |
| Light work | 200 | 8.0 | 33.5 | 280 | 12.0 | 12.0 | 7.2 | 3.8 | 11.4 | 5.6 | 40.0 | 0.4 | 160.0 | 9,000 | 1320 | 320 |
| Moderate work | 200 | 9.3 | 38.9 | 307 | 13.2 | 14.0 | 8.4 | 4.6 | 12.8 | 7.1 | 45.0 | 0.45 | 180.0 | 9,000 | 1320 | 360 |
| Hard work | 200 | 10.7 | 44.8 | 345 | 14.8 | 16.0 | 11.6 | 6.0 | 15.6 | 10.2 | 50.0 | 0.5 | 200.0 | 9,000 | 1320 | 400 |
| Pregnant mares <5 months | 200 | 6.7 | 28.1 | 252 | 10.8 | 8.0 | 5.6 | 3.0 | 10.0 | 4.0 | 40.0 | 0.4 | 160.0 | 12,000 | 1320 | 320 |
| Pregnant mares 11 months | 226 | 8.6 | 34 | 357 | 15.4 | 14.4 | 10.5 | 3.1 | 10.3 | 4.4 | 50.0 | 0.4 | 160.0 | 12,000 | 1320 | 320 |
| Lactating mares 1 month | 200 | 12.7 | 53.1 | 614 | 33.9 | 23.6 | 15.3 | 4.5 | 19.1 | 5.1 | 50.0 | 0.5 | 200.0 | 12,000 | 1320 | 400 |
| Lactating mares 6 month | 200 | 10.9 | 17.2 | 506 | 26.8 | 15.0 | 9.3 | 3.5 | 13.5 | 4.6 | 50.0 | 0.5 | 200.0 | 12,000 | 1320 | 400 |
| Foals 6 months | 86 | 6.2 | 26 | 270 | 11.6 | 15.5 | 8.6 | 1.7 | 5.2 | 2.0 | 21.6 | 0.22 | 86.4 | 3,900 | 1917 | 173 |
| Yearling 12 months | 128 | 7.5 | 31.4 | 338 | 14.5 | 15.1 | 8.4 | 2.2 | 7.0 | 2.8 | 32.1 | 0.39 | 155.0 | 7,000 | 2464 | 310 |
| 2 year old | 172 | 7.5 | 31.4 | 308 | 13.2 | 14.7 | 8.1 | 2.7 | 8.8 | 3.5 | 42.9 | 0.43 | 171.7 | 7,700 | 2352 | 343 |

# DAILY NUTRIENT REQUIREMENTS OF HORSES WEIGHING 400KG OR THOSE EXPECTED TO MATURE AT THIS WEIGHT

(Major nutrients from NRC *Nutrient Requirements of Horses* 2007)

| | Weight kg | DE Mcal | DE MJ | CP g | Lysine g | Ca g | P g | Mg g | K g | Na g | Cu mg | Se mg | Zn mg | Vit A IU | Vit D IU | Vit E IU |
|---|---|---|---|---|---|---|---|---|---|---|---|---|---|---|---|---|
| Adult maintenance average | 400 | 13.3 | 55.6 | 504 | 21.7 | 16.0 | 11.2 | 6.0 | 20.0 | 8.0 | 80.0 | 0.8 | 320.0 | 12,000 | 2640 | 400 |
| Light work | 400 | 16.0 | 67 | 559 | 24.1 | 24.0 | 14.4 | 7.6 | 22.8 | 11.1 | 80.0 | 0.8 | 320.0 | 18,000 | 2640 | 640 |
| Moderate work | 400 | 18.6 | 77.8 | 614 | 26.4 | 28.0 | 16.8 | 9.2 | 25.6 | 14.2 | 90.0 | 0.9 | 360.0 | 18,000 | 2640 | 720 |
| Hard work | 400 | 21.3 | 89.1 | 689 | 29.6 | 32.0 | 23.2 | 12.0 | 31.2 | 20.4 | 100.0 | 1.0 | 400.0 | 18,000 | 2640 | 800 |
| Very hard work | 400 | 27.6 | 115.5 | 804 | 34.6 | 32.0 | 23.2 | 12.0 | 42.4 | 32.8 | 100.0 | 1.0 | 400.0 | 18,000 | 2640 | 800 |
| Pregnant mares <5 months | 400 | 13.3 | 55.6 | 504 | 21.7 | 16.0 | 11.2 | 6.0 | 20.0 | 8.0 | 80.0 | 0.8 | 320.0 | 24,000 | 2640 | 640 |
| Pregnant mares 11 months | 453 | 17.1 | 71.5 | 714 | 30.7 | 28.8 | 21.0 | 6.1 | 20.7 | 8.8 | 100.0 | 0.8 | 320.0 | 24,000 | 2640 | 640 |
| Lactating mares 1 month | 400 | 25.4 | 106.3 | 1228 | 67.8 | 47.3 | 30.6 | 8.9 | 38.3 | 10.2 | 100.0 | 1.0 | 400.0 | 24,000 | 2640 | 800 |
| Lactating mares 6 month | 400 | 21.8 | 91.2 | 1012 | 53.5 | 30.0 | 18.6 | 7.0 | 27.0 | 9.2 | 100.0 | 1.0 | 400.0 | 24,000 | 2640 | 800 |
| Foals 6 months | 173 | 12.4 | 51.9 | 541 | 23.3 | 30.9 | 17.2 | 3.3 | 10.4 | 4.0 | 43.2 | 0.43 | 172.7 | 7,800 | 3834 | 345 |
| Yearling 12 months | 257 | 15.0 | 62.8 | 677 | 29.1 | 30.1 | 16.7 | 4.3 | 13.9 | 5.5 | 64.2 | 0.64 | 257.0 | 11,600 | 4471 | 514 |
| 2 year old | 343 | 15.0 | 62.8 | 616 | 26.5 | 29.3 | 16.3 | 5.3 | 17.6 | 7.0 | 85.8 | 0.86 | 343.4 | 15,500 | 4704 | 687 |

# DAILY NUTRIENT REQUIREMENTS OF HORSES WEIGHING 500KG OR THOSE EXPECTED TO MATURE AT THIS WEIGHT

(Major nutrients from NRC *Nutrient Requirements of Horses* 2007)

| | Weight kg | DE Mcal | DE MJ | CP g | Lysine g | Ca g | P g | Mg g | K g | Na g | Cu mg | Se mg | Zn mg | Vit A IU | Vit D IU | Vit E IU |
|---|---|---|---|---|---|---|---|---|---|---|---|---|---|---|---|---|
| Adult maintenance average | 500 | 16.7 | 70 | 630 | 27.1 | 20 | 14 | 7.5 | 25.0 | 10.0 | 100.0 | 1.0 | 400.0 | 15,000 | 3300 | 500 |
| Light work | 500 | 20 | 83.7 | 699 | 30.1 | 30 | 18 | 9.5 | 28.5 | 13.9 | 100.0 | 1.00 | 400.0 | 22,500 | 3300 | 800 |
| Moderate work | 500 | 23.3 | 97.5 | 768 | 33.0 | 35 | 21 | 11.5 | 32.0 | 17.8 | 100.0 | 1.13 | 450.0 | 22,500 | 3300 | 900 |
| Hard work | 500 | 26.6 | 111.3 | 862 | 37.1 | 40 | 29 | 15 | 39.0 | 25.5 | 125.0 | 1.25 | 500.0 | 22,500 | 3300 | 1000 |
| Very hard work | 500 | 34.5 | 144.4 | 1004 | 43.2 | 40 | 29 | 15 | 53.0 | 41.0 | 125.0 | 1.25 | 500.0 | 22,500 | 3300 | 1000 |
| Pregnant mares <5 months | 500 | 16.7 | 69.9 | 630 | 27.1 | 20.0 | 14.0 | 7.5 | 25.0 | 10.0 | 100.0 | 1.0 | 400.0 | 30,000 | 3300 | 800 |
| Pregnant mares 11 months | 566 | 21.4 | 89.6 | 893 | 38.4 | 36.0 | 26.3 | 7.7 | 25.9 | 11.0 | 125.0 | 1.0 | 400.0 | 30,000 | 3300 | 800 |
| Lactating mares 1 month | 500 | 31.7 | 132.6 | 1535 | 84.8 | 59.1 | 38.3 | 11.2 | 47.8 | 12.8 | 125.0 | 1.25 | 500.0 | 30,000 | 300 | 1000 |
| Lactating mares 6 month | 500 | 27.2 | 113.8 | 1265 | 66.9 | 37.4 | 23.2 | 8.7 | 33.7 | 11.5 | 125.0 | 1.25 | 500.0 | 30,000 | 3300 | 1000 |
| Foals 6 months | 216 | 15.5 | 64.9 | 676 | 29.1 | 38.6 | 21.5 | 4.1 | 13.0 | 5.0 | 54.0 | 0.54 | 215.9 | 9,700 | 4793 | 432 |
| Yearling 12 months | 321 | 18.8 | 78.7 | 846 | 36.4 | 37.7 | 20.9 | 5.4 | 17.4 | 6.9 | 80.3 | 0.8 | 321.2 | 14,500 | 5589 | 642 |
| 2 year old | 429 | 18.7 | 78.2 | 770 | 33.1 | 36.7 | 20.4 | 6.7 | 22.0 | 8.8 | 107.3 | 1.07 | 429.2 | 19,300 | 5880 | 858 |

# DAILY NUTRIENT REQUIREMENTS OF HEAVY HORSES WEIGHING 900 KG OR THOSE EXPECTED TO MATURE AT THIS WEIGHT

(Major nutrients from NRC *Nutrient Requirements of Horses 2007*)

| | Weight kg | DE Mcal | DE MJ | CP g | Lysine g | Ca g | P g | Mg g | K g | Na g | Cu mg | Se mg | Zn mg | Vit A IU | Vit D IU | Vit E IU |
|---|---|---|---|---|---|---|---|---|---|---|---|---|---|---|---|---|
| Adult maintenance average | 900 | 30.0 | 125.5 | 1134 | 48.8 | 36.0 | 25.2 | 13.5 | 45.0 | 18.0 | 180.0 | 1.8 | 720.0 | 27,000 | 5940 | 900 |
| Light work | 900 | 36.0 | 150.6 | 1259 | 54.1 | 54.0 | 32.4 | 17.1 | 51.3 | 25.0 | 180.0 | 1.8 | 720.0 | 40,500 | 5940 | 1440 |
| Moderate work | 900 | 42.0 | 175.8 | 1382 | 59.4 | 63.0 | 37.8 | 20.7 | 57.6 | 32.0 | 202.5 | 2.03 | 810.0 | 40,500 | 5940 | 1620 |
| Hard work | 900 | 48.0 | 200.9 | 1551 | 66.7 | 72.0 | 52.2 | 27.0 | 70.2 | 45.9 | 225.0 | 2.25 | 900.0 | 40,500 | 5940 | 1800 |
| Very hard work | 900 | 62.1 | 259.9 | 1808 | 77.7 | 72.0 | 52.2 | 27.0 | 95.4 | 73.8 | 225.0 | 2.25 | 900.0 | 40,500 | 5940 | 1800 |
| Pregnant mares <5 months | 900 | 30.0 | 125.5 | 1134 | 48.8 | 36.0 | 25.2 | 13.5 | 45.0 | 18.0 | 180.0 | 1.8 | 720.0 | 54,000 | 5940 | 1440 |
| Pregnant mares 11 months | 1019 | 38.5 | 161.1 | 1607 | 69.1 | 64.8 | 47.3 | 13.8 | 46.5 | 19.8 | 225.0 | 1.8 | 720.0 | 54,000 | 5940 | 1440 |
| Lactating mares 1 month | 900 | 54.4 | 227.7 | 2763 | 152.6 | 106.4 | 68.9 | 20.1 | 86.1 | 23.0 | 225.0 | 2.25 | 900.0 | 54,000 | 5940 | 1800 |
| Lactating mares 6 month | 900 | 46.3 | 193.7 | 2277 | 120.5 | 67.4 | 41.8 | 15.7 | 60.7 | 20.7 | 225.0 | 2.25 | 900.0 | 54,000 | 5940 | 1800 |
| Foals 6 months | 389 | 28.0 | 117.2 | 1217 | 52.3 | 69.5 | 38.7 | 7.5 | 23.3 | 9.1 | 97.1 | 0.97 | 388.6 | 17,500 | 8627 | 777 |
| Yearling 12 months | 578 | 33.8 | 141.5 | 1522 | 65.5 | 67.8 | 37.7 | 9.7 | 31.4 | 12.4 | 144.5 | 1.45 | 578.2 | 26,000 | 10061 | 1156 |
| 2 year old | 773 | 33.7 | 141 | 1386 | 59.6 | 66.0 | 36.7 | 12.0 | 39.6 | 15.8 | 193.1 | 1.93 | 772.6 | 34,800 | 10584 | 1545 |

In the USA, the NRC *Nutrient Requirements of Horses* is published by the National Research Council. These standards are statements of the nutrient requirements of various classes and weights of horses and are constantly revised and republished when required. Currently, following many years of research these published figures provide a high degree of accuracy. Although this is published in the USA it is used worldwide. Theses figures have been adapted from the 6th Edition published in 2007.

These figures assume feed intakes of 2.5% BW (bodyweight) for horses in hard work, lactating mares and growing youngstock, 2.25% BW for medium work and 2% BW for all others.

# Appendix 2
# Nutrient Composition of
# Selected Feedstuffs

All data in the tables of this appendix are reprinted with permission from the National Research Council (NRC), *Nutrient Requirements of Horses*, National Academies Press, Copyright 2007, National Academy of Sciences, Washington.

All values on a dry matter (DM) basis

| Feed | Type | DM % as fed | DE Mcal/ kg/DM | DE MJ/kg DM | CP % DM | Lys % DM | Oil % DM |
|---|---|---|---|---|---|---|---|
| Barley rolled | Conc. | 91.0 | 3.67 | 15.4 | 12.4 | 0.45 | 2.2 |
| Molassed sugar beet pulp 3% | Conc. | 88.0 | 2.84 | 11.9 | 10.0 | 0.42 | 1.1 |
| Unmolassed sugar beet pulp | Conc. | 88.3 | 2.8 | 11.7 | 10.0 | 0.44 | 1.1 |
| Brewers Grains dried | Conc. | 90.7 | 2.85 | 11.9 | 29.2 | 1.19 | 5.2 |
| Corn (maize) steam flaked | Conc. | 88.1 | 3.88 | 16.2 | 9.4 | 0.29 | 4.2 |
| Linseed meal solvent | Conc. | 90.3 | 2.85 | 11.9 | 32.6 | 1.2 | 1.7 |
| Molasses Sugar cane | Conc. | 74.3 | 4.06 | 17 | 5.8 | 0.06 | 0.2 |
| Oats rolled | Conc. | 90.0 | 3.27 | 13.7 | 13.2 | 0.55 | 5.1 |
| Oatfeed | Conc. | 90.0 | | 7.7 | 5.0 | 0.19 | 2.2 |
| Rice bran | Conc. | 90.6 | 3.35 | 14 | 15.5 | 0.72 | 15.2 |
| Peas | Conc. | | | 14.1 | 22.9 | 1.6 | 5.0 |
| Soybean Meal expellers | Conc. | 89.6 | 3.5 | 14.6 | 46.3 | 2.9 | 8.1 |
| Sunflower meal solvent | Conc. | 92.2 | 2.42 | 10.1 | 28.4 | 1.01 | 1.4 |
| Wheat Bran | Conc. | 89.1 | 3.22 | 13.5 | 17.3 | 0.7 | 4.3 |
| Wheatfeed | Conc. | 89.1 | 2.63 | 11.0 | 15.5 | 0.61 | 3.5 |
| Wheat Middlings | Conc. | 89.5 | 3.4 | 14.3 | 18.5 | 0.67 | 4.5 |

| | | DM % as fed | DE Mcal/ kg/DM | DE MJ/kg DM | CP % DM | Lys % DM | Oil % DM |
|---|---|---|---|---|---|---|---|
| Alfalfa meal 17%CP | Forage | 90.3 | 2.43 | 10.2 | 19.2 | 0.83 | 2.5 |
| High protein grass meal | Forage | 90.0 | 2.3 | 9.6 | 16.0 | 8.0 | 3.2 |
| Mostly Grass hay mature | Forage | 84.7 | 2.08 | 8.7 | 13.3 | 0.51 | 2.3 |
| Mostly Grass hay Mid mature | Forage | 87.3 | 2.19 | 9.2 | 17.4 | 0.68 | 2.6 |
| Mostly Grass hay Immature | Forage | 84.3 | 2.35 | 9.8 | 18.4 | 0.72 | 2.4 |
| Mostly Grass silage immature | Forage | 47.1 | 2.34 | 9.8 | 18.0 | 0.64 | 2.9 |
| Legume Hay Mid mature | Forage | 84.2 | 2.35 | 9.8 | 19.1 | 0.9 | 2.0 |
| Grass Haylage | Forage | 50–65 | 2.15 | 8–10 | 6–10 | – | – |
| Barley straw | Forage | 88.0 | 1.4 | 6.0 | 3.0 | 0 | 1.9 |
| Vegetable oil | High fat | 100.0 | 9.19 | 38.4 | 0 | 0 | 99.9 |

| NDF % DM | Ash % DM | Ca % DM | P % DM | Mg % DM | K% DM | Na % DM | Cu Mg/kg | Se Mg/kg | Zn Mg/kg |
|---|---|---|---|---|---|---|---|---|---|
| 20.8 | 2.9 | 0.06 | 0.39 | 0.14 | 0.56 | 0.02 | 6.0 | 0.11 | 38 |
| 44.4 | 7.4 | 0.89 | 0.09 | 0.23 | 1.11 | 0.35 | 11.3 | 0.14 | 22 |
| 45.8 | 7.3 | 0.91 | 0.09 | 0.23 | 0.96 | 0.31 | 11.0 | 0.14 | 22 |
| 47.4 | 4.3 | 0.3 | 0.67 | 0.26 | 0.5 | 0.04 | 11.0 | 1.06 | 85 |
| 9.5 | 1.5 | 0.04 | 0.3 | 0.12 | 0.42 | 0.02 | 3.0 | 0.07 | 27 |
| 36.1 | 6.5 | 0.4 | 0.83 | 0.55 | 1.22 | 0.09 | 19.0 | 1.05 | 69 |
| 0.4 | 13.3 | 1.0 | 0.1 | 0.42 | 4.01 | 0.22 | 66.0 | – | 21 |
| 30.0 | 3.3 | 0.11 | 0.4 | 0.16 | 0.52 | 0.03 | 8.0 | 0.48 | 41 |
| 63.5 | 7.0 | 0.8 | 1.2 | – | 7.0 | – | – | – | – |
| 26.1 | 10.4 | 0.07 | 1.78 | 0.81 | 1.57 | 0.03 | 10.0 | 0.17 | 71 |
| 17.2 | 2.7 | 0.7 | 4.0 | – | 11.0 | – | – | – | – |
| 21.7 | 5.5 | 0.36 | 0.66 | 0.3 | 2.12 | 0.04 | 17.0 | – | 72 |
| 40.3 | 7.7 | 0.48 | 1.0 | 0.63 | 1.5 | 0.04 | 32.0 | 0.5 | 88 |
| 42.5 | 6.3 | 0.13 | 1.18 | 0.53 | 1.32 | 0.04 | 11.0 | 0.5 | 85 |
| 31.0 | 5.0 | 1.0 | 10.0 | – | 12.0 | – | – | – | – |
| 36.7 | 5.0 | 0.16 | 1.02 | 0.42 | 1.38 | 0.03 | 10.0 | 0.46 | 91 |

| NDF % DM | Ash % DM | Ca % DM | P % DM | Mg % DM | K% DM | Na % DM | Cu Mg/kg | Se Mg/ kg | Zn Mg/kg |
|---|---|---|---|---|---|---|---|---|---|
| 41.6 | 11.0 | 1.47 | 0.28 | 0.29 | 2.37 | 0.1 | 9.0 | 0.36 | 28 |
| 54.0 | 7.0 | 6.0 | 2.3 | – | 21.0 | – | – | – | – |
| 62.5 | 7.9 | 0.73 | 0.27 | 0.21 | 2.09 | 0.1 | 8.0 | 0.09 | 24 |
| 55.1 | 9.5 | 0.88 | 0.36 | 0.25 | 2.45 | 0.01 | 9.0 | 0.09 | 26 |
| 49.6 | 9.2 | 1.01 | 0.31 | 0.26 | 2.83 | 0.03 | 9.0 | 0.12 | 24 |
| 49.9 | 9.1 | 1.02 | 0.34 | 0.25 | 2.88 | 0.03 | 9.0 | 0.11 | 28 |
| 47.2 | 9.1 | 1.17 | 0.3 | 0.27 | 2.34 | 0.08 | 9.0 | 0.15 | 24 |
| – | – | 5.1 | 1.8 | – | – | – | – | – | – |
| 64.0 | 7.0 | 2.0 | 0.4 | – | 19.0 | – | – | – | – |
| 0 | 0 | 0 | 0 | 0 | 0 | 0 | 0 | 0 | 0 |

# Appendix 3
# Modern Rules of Feeding

1. Feed horses according to bodyweight and monitor bodyweight every two weeks, adjusting feed intake accordingly.
2. Feed at least 1.0–1.5 lb (0.45–0.7 kg) of forage for each 100 lb (45 kg) of bodyweight. Total daily feed should be about 2.5–3.0 lb per 100 lb of bodyweight.
3. Feed horses according to the level of work or stage of the reproductive cycle
4. Assess horse's condition score for an accurate assessment of body condition
5. Feed good quality forage first and foremost, this should be long stemmed such as hay or haylage made specifically for horses and/or pasture, and do not leave without forage for longer than 4 hours.
6. Never feed mouldy forage/hay or feed or feed that has gone out of date.
7. Do not starve horses and ponies as this can result in serious health problems.
8. Store feed in proper conditions, dry and cool and vermin free.
9. Pay attention to hygiene keeping feed bins, buckets and mangers clean.
10. Feed little and often to mimic the horse's natural trickle feeding pattern.
11. Feed by weight not volume and weigh the feed contained in the scoop.
12. Do not feed more than 2 kg of concentrates at any one feed, for a 500 kg horse. If more is required add another feed during the day but space them out.
13. Do not feed a high starch concentrate feed to horses within 3 hours prior to exercise, feed forage or chaff instead.
14. Avoid sudden changes in diet – this includes concentrates and forage.

15. Make sure clean fresh water is always available, this is particularly important when horses are eating dry feeds or forage.
16. Check the manger for uneaten feed and adjust the ration if required.
17. Discard forage that has been trampled on the floor and left.
18. Avoid excess sugar and starch wherever possible.
19. Check horses' teeth regularly and maintain a good worming programme based upon anthelmintics (when required) and regular worm counts.
20. Provide free choice salt licks for all horses particularly if on forage only diets or on low levels of concentrates.
21. Do not mix balanced concentrate feeds with straights as this will unbalance the ration.
22. Add low energy high fibre chaffs to bulk out the feed for greedy horses.
23. Take care when adding supplements that they do not unbalance the feed.
24. Do not over-supplement horses, as this can be very dangerous.

# Appendix 4
# Conversion Factors

Some useful Conversion Factors

| Change value from | To | Multiply value by |
|---|---|---|
| acre | Square feet | 43,460 sqft/a |
| Square metre | Square feet | 10.76 sqft/sqm |
| g/kg | % | 0.1%/g/kg |
| mg/kg | % | 0.0001%/mg/kg |
| ppm | mg/kg | 1 mg/kg/ppm |
| ppm | mg/g | 0.001 mg/g/ppm |
| Kcal | kJ | 4.1855 kJ/Kcal |
| Mcal | Kcal | 1000 Kcal/Mcal |
| TDN kg | Kcal | 4409 Kcal/kg TDN |
| TDN lb | Kcal | 2000 Kcal/lb TDN |
| kg | lb | 2.2046 lb/kg |
| ounce | g | 28.35 g/oz |
| lb | kg | 0.4536 kg/lb |
| 1 ton | kg | 1000 kg/ton |
| 1 ton | lb | 2200 lb/ton |
| feet | cm | 30.48 cm/ft |
| Furlong | metres | 200 m/fu |
| hands | inches | 4 in/hand |
| Inch | cm | 2.54 cm/in |
| km | miles | 0.6214 miles/km |
| metres | feet | 3.281 ft/m |
| miles | feet | 5280 ft/mile |
| Miles/hr | Feet/min | 88 ft/min/mph |
| Farenheit | Centigrade or celcius | 5/9 (degrees F − 32) = degrees C |
| Centigrade or celcius | Farenheit | 9/5(degrees C + 32) = degrees F |
| litre | gallon | 0.2642 gal/l |
| ounce | millilitres ml | 29.57 ml/oz |
| pint | ounce | 16 oz/pint |
| pint | millilitres ml | 473 ml/pint |
| Teaspoon (1) | millilitres | 5 ml/tsp |

Metric measures, units SI symbols

| Name | SI unit | Symbol |
|---|---|---|
| Length | metre | m |
| Mass | kilogram | Kg |
| Energy | joule | J |

Metric unit prefixes

| Multiple | Prefix | Symbol | Submutltiple | Prefix | Symbol |
|---|---|---|---|---|---|
| $10^6$ | mega | M | $10^{-1}$ | deci | d |
| $10^3$ | kilo | k | $10^{-2}$ | centi | c |
| $10^2$ | hecto | h | $10^{-3}$ | milli | m |
| $10^1$ | deca | da | $10^{-6}$ | micro | u |
| | | | $10^{-9}$ | nano | n |
| | | | $10^{-12}$ | pico | p |

Therefore:

1 milligram (mg) is one thousandth of 1 gram
1 microgram (µg) is one millionth of 1 gram
1 g therefore is equal to 1000 mg
1 mg is equal to 1000 µg

Vitamins

| | Metric | IU (International Units) |
|---|---|---|
| Vitamin A | 800 mcg | 2400 |
| Vitamin D | 5 mcg | 200 |
| Vitamin E | 10 mg | 15 |

# Further Reading

ENUCO (2007)
*Applied Equine Nutrition and Training*
Wageningen Academic Publishers, The Netherlands

David Frape (2006)
Third Edition
*Equine Nutrition & Feeding*
Blackwell Publishing

Lon D. Lewis (1995)
*Equine Clinical Nutrition*
Williams & Wilkins

P McDonald, RA Edwards, JFD Greenhalgh (1992)
*Animal Nutrition*
Longman Scientific & Technical

National Research Council (2007)
*Nutrient Requirements of Horses*
National Academy of Sciences, Washington, USA

WG. Pond, DC. Church, KR Pond (1995)
*Basic Animal Nutrition and Feeding*
John Wiley & Sons, USA

54th Annual American Association of Equine Practitioners (AAEP) Convention (2008)

www.BEVA.org.uk

www.nutritionsociety.org

# Glossary

**Acidosis** – Increased acidity of the blood and decreased blood bicarbonate or decreased pH. Normal arterial blood pH 7.5.

**ADF (Acid detergent fibre)** – Term used in analysis of feedstuffs as a description of fibre including lignin cellulose and silica.

**Additive** – One or more ingredients added to a feed to fulfil a specific requirement often in very small amounts.

**Ad lib** (*ad libitum*) – Feed is offered free choice, i.e unrestricted. This is commonly applied to forage, but not under normal circumstances to concentrates unless referring to creep feeds for youngstock.

**Aerobic** – Aerobic respiration involves the breakdown of energy giving nutrients in the presence of oxygen from the lungs. This yields more energy.

**Alfalfa** (*see* **Lucerne,** *Medicago sativa*) – A legume commonly fed to horses, as hay or as a dried chaff. It is higher in protein.

**Alkalaemia** – Increased pH of the blood unrelated to changes in blood bicarbonate. Normal arterial blood pH is 7.5.

**Allergy** – A sensitivity, sometimes extreme, to a specific substance or feed either ingested or inhaled or through contact. This is normally a particular protein present in the feed. Allergic reactions or hypersensitivities are a result of the horse becoming sensitised to at least one antigen.

**Amines** – Compounds containing nitrogen. Thought to be involved in laminitis.

**Amino acid** – One of the 25 building blocks of proteins. These may be essential, i.e. must be supplied in the diet, or non-essential, i.e. the horse can synthesise them within the body.

**Anaerobic** – Anaerobic respiration involves the breakdown of energy giving nutrients in the absence of oxygen from the lungs. This yields less energy.

**Anorexia** – Loss of appetite, may be complete or partial.

**Antioxidant** – Helps to reduce the effects of harmful free radicals produced in the body from normal oxidation reactions.

**As fed** – Describes feed as it is given in its complete and natural state and not in terms of how much dry matter it contains.

**Ash** – The residue of food after burning at very high temperatures until the carbon fraction has been removed. It includes minerals and silica.

**Balanced** – This may apply to a feed, ration or diet. This term applies to the supply of all the nutrients required to meet requirements according to known published scientific data, e.g. NRC.

**Balancer** – A concentrated compound feed designed to be fed in smaller quantities often at a rate of approximately 500 g per day.

**Blocks** – Feed or mineral blocks. Compressed feed in a solid block or mass holding its shape, often molassed, offered to horses free choice.

**Botulism** – An often fatal disease affecting the nervous system caused by a toxin produced by the bacterium *Clostridium botulinum.* Botulism outbreaks have occurred in horses fed silage.

**Bruxism** – Grinding of the teeth.

**Buffers** – Substances that are able to maintain the pH (acidity or alkalinity).

**By-product** – Useful secondary products that are formed during manufacture of the main product.

**Calorie** – A unit of energy. Kilocalories or megacalories are more commonly used measurements in the USA for horses; in the UK kilojoules or megajoules are preferred.

**Carbohydrates** – Compounds composed of carbon, hydrogen and oxygen which include soluble CHOs such as sugars and starches and insoluble or structural CHOs such as cellulose and hemicellulose (fibre).

**Carriers** – An edible, often inert substance to which ingredients are added to aid mixing and extending for addition to horse feeds. Carriers are often used as a base for vitamin and mineral supplements.

**Cellulose** – The main structural carbohydrate of all plant cells constituting the fibre part of the horse's diet.

**Choke** – A blockage to the movement of food through the pharynx or oesophagus. This may be partial or complete and is often caused by dry impacted bulky feed. Horses with poor dentition are more prone to choke.

**Colic** – This refers to pain originating from the gut.

**Complete feed** – A compound feed designed to be fed as the sole feed, i.e. not requiring any additional food other than water.

**Compound feed** – Balanced, manufactured feed comprising a variety of ingredients, ground or otherwise processed, with additional nutrients to nutritionally balance the feed for a particular use. This could be a concentrate or fibre based chaff mix.

**Concentrate feed** – A feed containing a higher energy density or protein, or both, per given weight than forage. It is aimed at supplying additional concentrated nutrients to the total ration. Includes compound feeds, straights, oils and beet pulp.

**Corprophagy** – eating of droppings/faeces often seen in young foals.

**Cracked** – Feed, often straights, is mechanically crashed or crushed to aid digestion.

**Creatinine** – An excretory product found in horses' urine from the normal breakdown of muscle creatine. The amount produced is fairly constant for a given horse as it is related to muscle mass. Creatinine is therefore used to assess the excretion of other substances such as calcium, potassium and sodium in the creatinine clearance test.

**Creep feed** – A compound feed formulated specifically for foals to encourage them to eat compound feed and provide important nutrients that may otherwise be lacking in the pasture, for example. Creep feed is often offered free choice in special mangers which the only the foals have access to.

**Cribbing** – Refers to a vice whereby horses habitually swallow (*aerophagia*) air following latching their front teeth on to a horizontal gate/fence or stable door. This has been linked to gastric ulcers recently.

**Crude fibre** – An analytical term that describes the residue following chemical treatment in the lab; it encompasses cellulose, hemicellulose and lignin in the feed/forage tested.

**Cubes** – Compound feed that has been ground and often cooked before being forced through a die of a specific diameter. Cubes are otherwise known as nuts or pencils which tend to be larger than pellets.

**Decortication** – Also known as dehulling, the stripping off of the outer fibrous coat of husk/hull, by processing or mechanical means.

**Dehulling** – Also known as decortication, the stripping off of the outer fibrous coat of husk/hull, by processing or mechanical means.

**Dehydrated** – The process of removing water from a substance or excessive loss of water from the body.

**Diet** – All the food that the horse regularly consumes.

**Digestible energy (DE)** – Gross energy (GE) of a feedstuff minus the faecal energy (FE) results in the digestible energy (DE) measured in MJ/kg or Mcal/kg

**Distal** – Situated furthest from the point of attachment or origin, e.g. the distal end of a bone.

**Dry matter** – The remains following removal of water from the feed-stuff in an oven under laboratory conditions.

**Electrolytes** – Substances that become ions in solution and can conduct electricity. The balance of electrolytes in the horse's body is essential for normal function of cells and tissues. Electrolytes include sodium, potassium and chloride.

**Emulsify** – To break down fat droplets into smaller ones, thereby increasing surface area. Fats are emulsified in the digestive tract increasing the surface area for enzyme action.

**Epiphysitis** – A condition of youngstock whereby the growth plate or epiphysis become inflamed.

**Equine Metabolic Syndrome (EMS)** – A relatively new syndrome whereby the preliminary diagnosis is based on obesity, insulin resistance and sometimes onset of laminitis. EMS horses typically have fat deposits in the crest of the neck, over the tail head, above the eyes, behind the shoulders, and in the sheath of male horses. Diagnosis is confirmed by measuring insulin and glucose levels in the blood.

**Extruded/Extrusion** – The process by which feed is pushed through dies or holes under pressure causing rapid expansion of the feed.

**Feed** – Edible materials consumed by horses which supply energy, protein and other nutrients.

**Fines** – Material that passes through screens smaller than the dyes through which the feed has passed during manufacture of compound feeds.

**Forage** – Bulky food like grass, haylage or hay for browsing or grazing horses.

**Fortified** – Feed that has had vitamins and minerals added. It is usually in the form of a premix to balance the feed.

**Founder** – Laminitis, a very painful serious health problem affecting one of more hooves, usually both front hooves.

**Gelatinisation** – Usually refers to the physical breakdown or rupture of starch grains in cereals following treatment with some combination of heat, moisture and pressure during feed manufacture.

**Glucagon** – A hormone produced by the pancreas, which is released when blood glucose level is low (hypoglycaemia), causing the liver to convert stored glycogen into glucose and release it into the blood-stream. The action of glucagon is opposite to that of insulin.

**Glucogenic** – A substance that may produce glucose.

**Gluconeogenesis** – The production of glucose from amino acids within the body cells.

**Gluten** – A tough viscid substance remaining following washing of flour from grain to remove starch. Gluten, for example, gives dough its stickiness.

**Glycolysis** – A major biochemical pathway whereby glucose is chemically broken down to produce energy in the first of a two stage process within the body cells.

**Grain** – The seeds of cereal plants including oats, barley and maize or corn.

**Haylage** – Haylage is a fermented ensiled forage that is usually a grass mix with a higher dry matter than silage but lower than hay.

**Herbage** – Succulent herbaceous vegetation such as green leafy plants as found in pasture.

**Hindgut** – The posterior part of the horse's digestive tract which includes the caecum, large colon and small colon otherwise known as the large intestine. This is the main area of fermentation of fibre.

**Hulls** – The outer covering of grain or peas and beans. From Old English 'hulu' meaning husk.

**Husk** – The dry outer covering of some grains.

**Hydrolysis** – Hydrolysis is a chemical reaction or process in which a chemical compound is broken down by reaction with water. This is the type of reaction that is used to break down storage carbohydrates such as glycogen. Water is added in this reaction.

**Hyper-** – Prefix signifying a greater quantity or amount, e.g. hyperglycaemia (high blood sugar).

**Hypo-** – Prefix signifying a smaller amount or quantity, e.g. hypoglycaemia (low blood sugar).

**Insulin** – Insulin is a hormone secreted from the pancreas when blood sugar levels are increased, causing liver and muscle cells to take in glucose and store it in the form of glycogen, and causing fat cells to take in blood lipids and turn them into triglycerides. In addition it has several other anabolic effects throughout the horse's body.

**Insulin Resistance** – This is when cells become resistant to the glucose uptake action of insulin. Initially, this means that more insulin is needed (hyperinsulinaemia) to keep blood glucose concentrations within normal limits after a starchy or high sugar feed.

**International Unit (IU)** – An international agreed unit of vitamin potency. This is a unit of measurement for the amount of a vitamin substance, based on measured biological activity or effect.

**Kibbling** – Crushed or cracked feed that has been cooked prior to the extrusion process.

**Legume** – A legume is a plant from the family *Leguminosae* or a fruit of these plants. Well known legumes include alfalfa, clover, peas and soya beans. Legumes are able to fix atmospheric nitrogen, owing to a symbiotic relationship with certain bacteria found in the root nodules of these plants. They therefore tend to be higher in protein.

**Lipase** – Lipases perform essential roles in the digestion, transport and processing of dietary lipids (e.g. triglycerides, fats, oils) in horses.

**Lucerne (*Medicago sativa*)** – A legume commonly fed to horses, as hay and/or as a dried chaff. It is higher in protein than most pasture plants.

**Lysine** – Lysine is an essential amino acid required in the horse's diet.

**Macrominerals** – Minerals required in larger quantities including calcium, phosphorus and sodium.

**Macronutrients** – The nutrients consumed in the largest quantities, e.g. water, carbohydrates, proteins and fats.

**Metabolism** – This refers to all the chemical reactions that occur in all living organisms in order to maintain life. These processes allow horses to grow and reproduce, maintain their structures, and respond to their environments. Metabolism is usually divided into two categories. Catabolism breaks down organic matter, for example to harvest energy in cellular respiration. Anabolism, on the other hand, uses energy to build components of cells such as proteins.

**Microminerals** – Minerals required in tiny or minute quantities otherwise known as trace minerals including copper, selenium, and zinc.

**Micronisation** – A feed manufacturing process which cooks cereals and peas under infrared burners. This results in a rapid rise in internal temperature of the grain thereby gelatinising the starch making it more digestible.

**Micronutrients** – Nutrients required in smaller amounts such as vitamins and minerals.

**Middlings** – By-product of the flour milling process that is graded according to the proportion of bran, germ and endosperm.

**Mitochondrion** – Membrane enclosed cell organelle (part of the cell) that is often referred to as the power house of the cell.

**Monensin** – An antibiotic used extensively in the beef and dairy industries to improve growth rates, where it is marketed under the name Rumensin. Monensin is extremely toxic and can be fatal when fed to horses.

**Mycotoxins** – Toxins produced by fungi. Mycotoxins vary considerably in their severity and effects on the horse's health.

**Neutral Detergent Fibre (NDF)** – This has been widely accepted as a determinant for dietary fibre in forage and cereal grains as it estimates the content of cellulose, hemicellulose and lignin present.

**Nutrient** – Any substance that can be metabolised by an animal to give energy and build tissue or provide nourishment.

**Oxalate** – A substance that can combine with calcium preventing digestion and absorption in the gut. Consumption of oxalates by grazing horses may result in kidney disease.

**Pellets** – Compound feed formed by forcing compacted, ground, often cooked ingredients through a die to produce pellets. Pellets are smaller than cubes.

**Peristalsis** – The rhythmic contraction of smooth muscle pushing ingested food along the digestive tract.

**Phosphagens** – High energy storage compounds mainly found in equine muscle tissue, e.g. creatine phosphate.

**Phytates** – The principal storage form of phosphorus in plants, particularly in bran and grains. Phosphorus is generally not bioavailable to horses as they lack phytase the enzyme required to break down phytate.

**Prebiotics** – Non-digestible (by the horse) feed ingredients that beneficially affect the horse by selectively stimulating the growth and/or activity of certain beneficial bacteria in the hindgut. Fructo-oligosaccharides are an example of prebiotics.

**Premix** – A mixture of minerals and vitamins and other ingredients, often in a carrier that is mixed into compound feed during the manufacturing process to balance the feed for the purpose for which it is intended, i.e. to meet nutrient requirements.

**Probiotics** – Dietary supplements containing potentially beneficial bacteria or yeasts. Strains of the genera *Lactobacillus* and *Bifidobacterium* are the most widely used probiotic bacteria. Probiotic bacterial cultures are intended to assist the horse's naturally occurring gut flora to re-establish themselves in the horse's hindgut.

**Protease** – Any of various enzymes that bring about the breakdown of proteins into peptides or amino acids by hydrolysis. The digestive enzyme pepsin is an example of a protease.

**Protein** – A large molecule composed of one or more chains of amino acids in a specific order.

**Proteolysis** – Digestion of proteins by cellular enzymes called proteases or by intramolecular digestion.

**Proximal** – Situated nearest to point of attachment or origin, e.g. the proximal end of a bone.

**Quidding** – The dropping of small amounts of feed from the horse's mouth during chewing, most often as a result of sharp teeth or damage to the mouth or tongue.

**Ration** – The amount of feed given daily to the horse.

**Rolling** – Mechanically breaking up cereals during feed manufacture by running the cereal ingredients through large rollers.

**Roughage** – Describes fibrous feeds such as hay, haylage and straw.

**Self-fed** – Feed is offered free choice, i.e unrestricted. This is commonly applied to forage, but not under normal circumstances to concentrates unless referring to creep feeds for youngstock.

**Silage** – This is a fermented, ensiled, low dry matter forage such as grass or maize usually fed to ruminants.

**Steaming** – Use of steam during the feed manufacturing process, which helps to improve starch digestibility.

**Straights** – Single cereal feeds are often referred to as straights and include oats, barley, maize or corn, soya bean and also bran (wheat and rice).

**Supplement** – A substance added in small amounts, usually daily, to "improve" the nutrient value of the overall diet, such as vitamins and minerals. May include probiotics, prebiotics and nutraceuticals such as herbs, glucosamine, chondroitin and MSM (methyl sulphonyl methane).

**Trace minerals** – Minerals required in tiny or minute quantities otherwise known as trace minerals including copper, selenium, and zinc.

**Water soluble carbohydrates** – Soluble compounds including monosaccharides, disaccharides, oligosaccharides and fructans.

# Index

α-amylase, 20
acid detergent fibre (ADF), 137
adenosine triphosphate (ATP), 67, 86
aerobic system, 90,
alfalfa (lucerne), 53, 110
alkali disease, 75,
aloe vera, 142
amine group, 43
amino acids, 42, 114
amylopectin, 38, 114
amylase, 38, 114
anaemia, 72
anaerobic system, 91
antioxidants, 52, 57, 204
arabinose, 34
arabinoxylans, 40
autotrophic nutrition, 2

ß-carotene, 52
B complex vitamins, 58, 84, 206
balancers, 126
barley, 117
  boiling, 118
bicarbonate, 19
bile, 19, 20
bilirubin, 20
biliverdin, 20
biological molecules, 27
bioplex minerals, 77
biotin, 58
blocks feed/mineral, 129, 130
bodyweight

assessment, 153
botulism, 108
bran (wheat), 118
branch chain amino acids (BCAA),
    44, 205
breeding stock, 171
brewers grains, 124
brewers yeast, 76
Bruner's glands, 19
butyric acid, 41

caecum, 6, 22
calcitonin, 64
calcitrol, 54
calcium
   homeostasis, 65
   serum calcium, 66
calcium to phosphorus ratio, 67
carbohydrates, 1, 2, 27, 28, 31, 58,
    115, 177
carotenoids, 52
cellulase, 11
cellulose 6, 11, 22, 39
cereal grains, 114
   by-products, 120
   processing, 119
cereal starch, 20, 39
chaff, 110
chelated minerals, 77
chloride, 69
choke, 198
cholecalciferol, 53